W0228013

Springer-Verlag Italia Srl.

L. Allegra • F. Blasi (Eds)

Mechanisms
and Management
of COPD Exacerbations

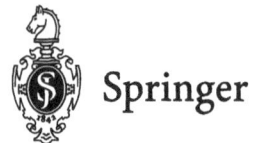 Springer

LUIGI ALLEGRA
FRANCESCO BLASI
Institute of Respiratory Diseases
University of Milan
IRCCS Ospedale Maggiore
Milan, Italy

The Editors and Authors wish to thank SmithKline Beecham S.p.A. for the support and help in the realization of this volume

© Springer-Verlag Italia 2000
Originally published by Springer-Verlag Italia, Milano in 2000

ISBN 978-88-470-0066-7   ISBN 978-88-470-2115-0 (eBook)
DOI 10.1007/978-88-470-2115-0

Library of Congress Cataloging-in-Publication data:

Mechanisms and management of COPD exacerbations / [edited by] L. Allegra, F. Blasi.
    p. cm.
    Includes bibliographical references and index.
    ISBN
    1. Lungs--Diseases, Obstructive. 2. Lungs–Diseases, Obstructive–Complications. I.
Allegra, Luigi. II. Blasi, F.

RC776.O3 M43 1999
616.2'4–dc21

99-012497

Cover design: Simona Colombo, Milan
Typesetting and layout: Graphostudio, Milan

SPIN: 10744177

Table of Contents

Chronic Bronchitis and Its Exacerbations: Definitions and Evaluations

L. ALLEGRA, F. BLASI

In the year 2000, it is rather uncommon for the definition of a disease to be uncertain or crude. It is even more surprising for a definition to be left unchanged for over 40 years notwithstanding its mediocrity.

Such is the case for the current definition of chronic bronchitis (CB) that dates back to the early 1960s [1]: "presence of cough and expectoration on most days during at least 3 consecutive months for not less than 2 consecutive years, in patients in whom other causes of chronic cough such as infection with *Mycobacterium tuberculosis*, carcinoma of the lung, chronic heart failure, bronchiectasis, cystic fibrosis, etc. have been excluded." This definition is excessively open to individual interpretation and has few elements that allow a quantitative evaluation of the disease. Moreover, the definition applies both to so-called simple CB or "des gros troncs" [2] as Galy named it (functionally determined solely by increased airway resistance) and to obstructive CB. The latter presents pathological phenomena involving bronchioles and alveoli (and the relative clinical and functional consequences) and is the basis for the devastating and often progressive affection defined as chronic obstructive pulmonary disease (COPD).

So modest has the definition appeared, that during the term as president of the Societas Europaea Pneumologiae in 1985, Allegra proposed the gathering of 10 experts, including 8 from European countries and one each from the United States and Canada, chosen among those that the literature indicated to be leaders in the field. The result was that the previously mentioned definition was considered to be criticizable but could not be improved.

Similarly criticizable is the definition proposed by Anthonisen et al. in 1987 [3] for acute exacerbations of chronic bronchitis (AECB), although it cannot be considered definitive and fully codified [4]. The "major" criterion ("Winnipeg I") for AECB was defined by a triad: increased sputum volume, increase in its purulence, and increase in dyspnea. Furthermore, two additional "minor" criteria were considered, defined by the presence of 2 of 3, or only 1 of 3 of the above manifestations (Winnipeg II and III, respectively). Leaving aside the modesty of this definition, which probably adds further coarseness to that of CB, we would like to underline its main inconsistencies:

Institute of Respiratory Diseases, University of Milan, IRCCS Ospedale Maggiore, Milan, Italy

a) The word "increase", referred to the three Winnipeg variables is excessively vague, since 10%-20% increases must not be placed on the same level of severity with 100% increases. The use of numerical scores, whenever possible, appears mandatory. This would be a decided step forward since numerical scores are currently available for a quantitative evaluation of sputum quantity, dyspnea, and possibly for purulence also, irrespective of the associated microscopical examination.

b) Among the major criteria for the definition of AECB there is no mention of cough, one of the few central elements in the definition of chronic bronchitis. It is, however, unthinkable that acute exacerbations may develop in the absence of an increase in this main feature. In a recent symposium among 70 leading Italian pulmonologists, a vast majority expressed the opinion that cough must be given high consideration, and this concept was underscored by the opinion of roughly 2000 practitioners. Specifically, the former indicated that immediately following sputum volume, increase in cough was the leading characteristic defining the presence of an exacerbation in CB patients [5]. Unfortunately, cough characteristics are still elusive in terms of qualitative evaluation, notwithstanding the presence of sonographic recordings (currently too expensive) capable of determining (quantitatively, on the basis of mathematical parameters) the number of coughs over time, and their duration (in milliseconds), frequency (Hz), and sonority (decibels).

c) The Anthonisen triad includes dyspnea (Appendix I), thus encompassing among the Winnipeg I criteria only obstructive CB. This ambiguity leads to serious difficulties in performing multicentric trials on just exacerbated CB.

d) Without the aid of a microscope (according to the criteria of Bartlett et al. [6], Appendix II), the appreciation of purulence and its variations is no easy task. In the previously mentioned meeting among Italian experts, in an attempt to overcome this difficulty (as may be performed by applying the Cumming and Semple criteria [7], Appendix III), a favorable opinion was expressed for evaluation of sputum color variations as an indication of sputum purulence [5]. Our group performed studies in this direction by devising a "colorimetric stick" with the 10 most common "average colors" obtained with approximately 50 color shades evaluated on over 500 sputum samples [8, Appendix IV].

e) The daily secretion output would be easily obtainable if the patient could expectorate all day into a jar, but this is evidently rendered impossible in the normal performance of daily activities. To overcome this practical difficulty it has been suggested that recording of 24-hour overall sputum production may be substituted by assessment of sputum production over the first hour following awakening, a time generally spent in the home, making sputum collection more comfortable and "private" for the patient. A statistically significant correlation was observed between sputum quantity during the first hour following awakening and overall 24-hour quantity [8].

We therefore feel that the use of numerical elements defining the single features of AECB should be improved and encouraged, resorting to adjectives (e.g. scarce, moderate, or abundant; worse, equal, or better) or prevalence signs (e.g. +, ++, +++; ↑, ↑↑, ↑↑↑) only where numerical parameters are not available. We hope that consensus may be reached not only on a better definition of AECB, but also on creating and validating a reliable symptom score that may be employed both in single patient evaluations and, more importantly, in trials on treatment efficacy. Previous experiences, including our own, on the possible use of symptom scores were highly satisfactory [9-11].

Appendix I Degrees of dyspnea [9, 10]

0, No dyspnea
1, Dyspnea on walking uphill or up 2 flights of stairs
2, Dyspnea when walking at a rapid pace, or after 1 flight of stairs, or when walking slightly uphill
3, Dyspnea while walking on a road or in a garden at ground level
4, Dyspnea while moving about in the home or while performing personal hygiene activities
5, Dyspnea at rest

Appendix II Microscopic evaluation of the purulent component within sputum samples, according to Bartlett et al. [6]. Samples with > 25 epithelial cells per microscopic field are considered not appropriate for culture. Specimens with scores 4-6 are appropriate for culture

	Composition [cells/microscopic field (x 100)]	
Purulence score	Squamous epithelial cells	Neutrophils
1	> 25	< 10
2	> 25	10-25
3	> 25	> 25
4	10-25	> 25
5	> 10	> 25
6	< 25	> 25

Appendix III Nonmicroscopic evaluation of sputum purulence, according to Cumming and Semple [7]. The specimen must be examined fresh, immediately following expectoration, in a transparent container, against a dark background

Sputum purulence	Sputum characteristics
Mucous sputum	Colorless, absence of pus
Mucopurulent sputum	Traces of pus[a]
	0%-25%
	25%-50%
	< 75%
Purulent sputum	Almost completely formed by pus

[a] Saliva gives sputum a foamy appeareance and compromises the determination of the quantitative mucus/pus ratio. However, saliva is not the only cause of foam within sputum samples: presence of foam in the absence of saliva may be a sign of improvement following antibiotic treatment

Appendix IV

We analyzed the colors of 573 sputum samples by comparing them with the colors of a multicolor "ink catalogue" (gamma "Pantone"). The ink catalogue was chosen so that the selected colors could be easily printed without having to resort to quadrichromy printing techniques, which are very limited and nearly ineffective. All colors in sputum samples were in the catalogue. It was only necessary to resort to a blend of colors for the definition of "white" in mucous sputum.

We identified about 50 different colors, including shades or tones of individual colors. For practical reasons we selected 10 reference colors together with a "physiological" white. In addition to being the most commonly occurring ones, these 10 colors were used as reference "average" colors for other shades and tones (Fig. 1).

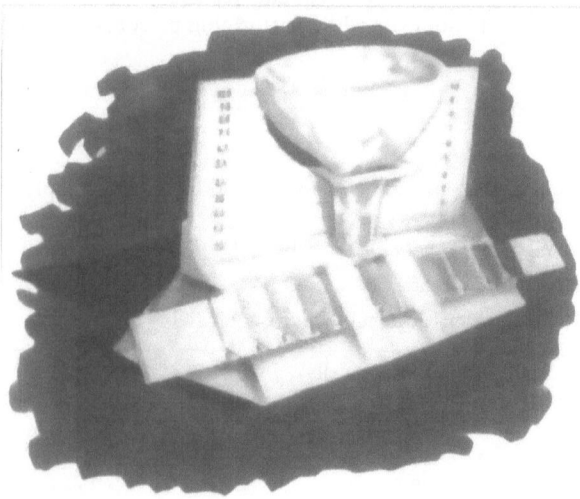

Fig. 1. A tool for performing a quick color test on sputum. The colorimetric scale slides under the funnel filled with the secretion, thereby allowing the approximate color identification. Each color is coded with a number, which can be compared, later, with other sputum samples

Defining a color according to a colorimetric stick provides a better approximation than describing a color as "yellowish", "whitish", or "greenish", etc. In a pilot study we found that patients are often very imprecise in identifying colors: what is described as yellow is often, in fact, green, and white is often actually gray. We were able to overcome this difficulty by furnishing an "official" reference color by sliding a colorimetric stick along the tube containing the specimen being examined and reading the number corresponding to that color.

References

1. Meneely GR, Renzetti AD, Steele JD, Wyatt JR, Harris HW (1962) Chronic bronchitis, asthma and pulmonary emphysema. A statement of the Committee on Diagnostic Standards for Non-tuberculous Respiratory Diseases. Am Rev Respir Dis 85:762-768
2. Galy P, Loire R (1967) L'emphysème pulmonaire diffus et la bronchite chronique. Etude anatomique. Corrélations anatomo-radiologiques, anatomo-fonctionnelles, anatomo-cliniques. Bull Physio-path Respir 3:179-236

3. Anthonisen NR, Manfreda J, Warren CPW, Hershfield ES, Harding GKM, Nelson NA (1987) Antibiotic therapy in exacerbations of chronic obstructive pulmonary disease. Ann Intern Med 106:196-204

4. Ball P (1995) Epidemiology and treatment of chronic bronchitis and its exacerbations. Chest 108:43s-52s

5. Grassi V (1997) Definizione, storia naturale, etiologia. In: Allegra L, Donner C, Blasi F, Lusuardi M (eds) Riacutizzazione di bronchite cronica. Edizioni Multimed, Milano, pp 7-15

6. Bartlett JG, Brewe NS, Ryan KJ, Washigton JA (1978) Laboratory diagnosis of lower respiratory tract infection. Cumitech 7, Am Soc Microb 1-15

7. Cumming G, Semple SJ (1973) Disorders of the respiratory system. Blackwell, London

8. Allegra L, Blasi F, Diano PL, Fasano V, Tarsia P, Valenti V (2000) Modello per la valutazione delle riacutizzazioni nel paziente bronchitico cronico. Giorn Ital Mal Tor 54:221-228

9. Allegra L, Bonsignore G, Cresci F, Fumagalli G, Mandelli V, Morpurgo M, Panuccio P, Pasargiklian M, Rampulla C, Viroli L (1979) Classificazione del deficit respiratorio nelle broncopneumopatie croniche ostruttive: proposta di nomogrammi. Minerva Pneumol 18:197-218

10. Allegra L, Bonsignore G, Cresci F, Fumagalli G, Mandelli V, Morpurgo M, Panuccio P, Pasargiklian M, Rampulla C, Viroli L (1984) Classification of respiratory functional impairment in chronic obstructive pulmonary disease. Respiration 45:175-184

11. Allegra L, Grassi C, Grossi E, Pozzi E, Blasi F, Frigerio D, Nastri A, Montanari C, Montanari M, Serra G (1991) Ruolo degli antibiotici nel trattamento delle riacutizzazioni della bronchite cronica: risultati di uno studio italiano multicentrico. Giorn Ital Mal Tor 45:138-148

COPD Epidemiology and Natural History

L. Allegra[1], P. Tarsia[2]

Introduction

Since the 1950s numerous consensus statements have been issued in the attempt to reach rational definitions and uniform terminology of diseases involving the lower airways [1-7]. These definitions represent a mixture of clinical, pathological and functional descriptions. The terms "chronic bronchitis" and "emphysema" date further back in time and are widely accepted. By the 1820s emphysema had been well defined, clearly described, and recognised to be common. The diagnosis of chronic bronchitis was first applied in 1805 to patients with chronic cough, breathlessness, and recurrent exacerbations during winter months. Conversely, a variety of definitions have been put forward to incorporate the concept of obstruction to airflow and chronic sputum production. Among these, "chronic obstructive pulmonary disease" (COPD) is certainly the most widely accepted.

In the 1995 European Respiratory Society (ERS) Consensus Statement, COPD was defined as "a disorder characterised by reduction of maximum expiratory flow and forced emptying of the lungs; features that do not change markedly over several months. Most of the airflow is slowly progressive and irreversible. The airflow limitation is due to varying combinations of airways disease and emphysema; the relative contribution of the two processes is difficult to define in vivo" [5].

COPD is an all-inclusive and non-specific term that refers to a defined set of breathing-related symptoms [5, 6]: chronic cough, expectoration, varying degrees of exertional dyspnoea, and a significant progressive reduction in expiratory airflow. It is therefore an umbrella term used to encompass several more specific respiratory diagnoses that may occur individually or in combination.

[1] Institute of Respiratory Diseases, University of Milan, IRCCS Ospedale Maggiore, Milan, Italy;
[2] Division of Emergency Medicine, IRCCS Ospedale Maggiore, Milan, Italy

The majority of patients are aged over 50 years, have been smokers for many years, and report symptoms such as dyspnoea on exertion, wheezing specifically with a cold, and often chronic productive cough. Clinically the diagnosis is based on a combination of lung function values and clinical symptoms. The prevalence of symptoms and lung function impairment increases with age, particularly in smokers who do not refrain from smoking [8, 9].

Epidemiology

In the United States, COPD is the fourth leading cause of death after heart disease, cancer, and stroke [10], killing more patients than does diabetes mellitus. Prevalence and mortality have been increasing steadily in contrast to many other leading chronic diseases [11]. Given the overall increase in life expectancy, greater prevalence and mortality from COPD may be expected in the future.

In epidemiological studies, the degree of irreversible lung functional impairment required to define COPD is < 1.64 residual standard deviations below predicted for major respiratory parameters (FEV_1 < 70% predicted and FEV_1/VC ratio 11% below predicted) [5]. Prevalence rates are generally expressed with reference to the overall general population (age range, 15-95 years). Considering that the disease predominantly affects middle-aged to elderly smokers, true epidemiological impact in relevant population subsets may be grossly underestimated.

Both chronic bronchitis and emphysema are important causes of restricted activity, chronic disability, and lost productivity. Overall costs in the US in 1993 were estimated at $14.7 billion for medical expenses, $6.1 billion for hospital care, $4.4 billion for professional services, $2.5 billion for drugs, $1.5 billion for nursing home care, and $1.0 billion for home care [12].

The major difficulty in obtaining reliable epidemiological data regarding chronic obstructive pulmonary disease is related to the fact that COPD is not a clearly standardised diagnosis. The confusion in terminology has led to problems in defining the incidence of COPD. In Britain, the combination of chronic cough and expectoration, dyspnoea, and airflow obstruction has traditionally been labelled as chronic bronchitis [13], whereas in the US there has been a tendency to refer to this as emphysema. Three decades ago, the use of these different terminologies gave the impression that the death rate from "chronic bronchitis" was approximately 40 times that in the Unites States [14]. COPD does not in fact appear as a specific single disease category in any revision of the International Classification of Disease (ICD) system, although subgroups including "chronic bronchitis" (Code 491) and "emphysema" (Code 492) are present. However, a category of "chronic airway obstruction not elsewhere classified" was introduced into the ninth revision of the ICD, issued in 1979 [15]. Among causes of death, the rubric "chronic obstructive pulmonary diseases and allied conditions" (Codes 490-496) encompasses deaths due to asthma, bronchiectasis, and extrinsic allergic alveolitis in addition to chronic bronchitis and emphysema.

Morbidity

Information on COPD morbidity can be obtained from a wide variety of sources (self-reports, hospital admissions, general practitioner consultations, etc.) in many countries but is nonetheless flawed by the previously mentioned difficulties in diagnostic standardisation.

Data from the 1993 National Health Interview Survey in the US, based on self-reported conditions, indicate that 13.8 million Americans have chronic bronchitis and 2 million have emphysema [16]. Considering that up to 50% of cases may be undiagnosed and therefore unreported, COPD may be present in > 30 million patients. The prevalence of chronic bronchitis in the general population has apparently increased from 3.3% in 1970 to 5.4% in 1993 [16, 17]. Similar results were recorded in Europe by a Dutch group who found significant increases in COPD and asthma prevalence between 1977 and 1992 in the same geographical area [18]. There are apparently no marked age or sex differences in time trends for the prevalence of chronic bronchitis, whereas the prevalence of emphysema is much higher in men than in women, and in whites than in blacks [11, 16, 17]. In the three-year period 1986-1989, COPD was responsible for 114 million days of restricted activity annually, thus ranking among the 10 highest chronic conditions in the United States [19].

Mortality

Mortality data from the US demonstrate a relatively persistent overall increase in COPD mortality over a 35-year period between 1950 and 1985 [20]. Over this period the overall COPD mortality increased approximately four-fold. Mortality figures recorded in England and Wales between 1971 and 1990 indicate a relatively static overall COPD mortality during the study period [21].

The international variability in COPD mortality is an area of great interest. Data collected by the World Health Organization indicate marked variations in the overall mortality from COPD in different countries, ranging between the extremes of > 400 deaths per 100 000 in Romania to < 100 per 100 000 in Japan [22]. International differences may be explained by differing exposure (smoking habits, environmental pollutants), genetic susceptibility, and rate of respiratory infections.

Approximately 95% of COPD mortality occurs in subjects aged over 55 years [23]. The age-adjusted death rate for COPD is 60% higher in men than in women and appears to change over time [10]. During the 1960s increases in mortality rates were much greater in men than in women [11]. However, by the 1980s the increase was strikingly greater in women than in men and greater at older rather than younger ages. Mortality in men aged 65-74 years has since leveled off but continues to increase in women aged over 55 and men over 75 [11]. Mortality trends largely reflect the variations in exposure to cigarette smoking for different age cohorts. Relatively high mortality rates among elderly men may be explained by the massive exposure to cigarette smoking in men born between 1910 and 1940 [24]. The increase in mortality in middle-aged females may be associated with increased cigarette consumption.

The precise determination of COPD mortality is limited by the frequent confusion in the classifications present on death certificates [25]. For example, COPD may be absent on death certificates in 80% of cases where clinical history suggests this diagnosis [20, 25]. Further problems arise from the ICD categories. Inspection in COPD mortality trends over time suggests that in more than one country there has been considerable diagnostic transfer from the chronic bronchitis to the chronic airway obstruction category since the latter was introduced in 1979 [21].

Overall data therefore indicate that in most developed countries COPD is one of the major causes of death, particularly in older age groups, and more so in males than females.

Risk Factors

Cigarette Smoking

Cigarette smoking is by far the most important contributor to the development of COPD. Clinical studies have shown that among non-smokers the disease is very rare [26, 27]. Incidence in pipe and cigar smokers lies somewhere in between [28]. The duration and intensity of cigarette smoking are of equal importance in calculating a dose-response, factors that can be combined into a single index by calculating the number of pack-years (packages of 20 cigarettes/day x years smoked) [29].

Up to the start of the twentieth century, cigarette smoking was rather unusual: chewing tobacco or pipe smoking accounted for most tobacco consumption. Cigarette smoking increased rapidly among males since World War I [30]. Among females, the incidence of smoking increased later on, following World War II [30]. Between 1900 and 1960 cigarette consumption per person in the United States crept from 41 to 3888 per year [31]. From the 1960s, cigarette smoking started to decline in both sexes.

Tobacco smoke is a complex mixture of more than 100 volatile and particulate chemical substances, and it is not known which of these components are responsible for the increased susceptibility to COPD. The tar content alone is insufficient to define an accurate measure of the potential effect of toxic components on the airways of smokers [32].

Numerous studies conducted world-wide have shown that cigarette smoking is the principal determinant of airway obstruction. This has been shown in both cross-sectional prevalence studies and longitudinal prospective studies [29, 32-37]. In cross-sectional studies, FEV_1 levels decreased with increasing amount of smoking [32], and the influence of smoking on lung function may be detected at as early as age 20 years [29]. Perhaps the best known longitudinal study is that conducted by Fletcher, et al. in the 1960s in London [33]. This study demonstrated that non-smokers show a gradual decline in FEV_1 with age, and smokers who are not susceptible to the effects of cigarette smoke show a similar, although somewhat accelerated decline. Individuals who are susceptible to cigarette smoke and who smoke regularly demonstrate an accelerated decline in FEV_1 which increases in rapidity with increasing age (the "horse race effect") [34]. Smoking cessation has been shown in many studies to result in normalisation of decline in FEV_1 to the rate of never smokers [34-36]. A four-decade prospective observation of mortality in relation to smoking in British male doctors was completed in the 1990s [37]. This study showed that the overall COPD mortality was 7-times greater among "light" smokers (1-14 cigarettes/day) than non-smokers. Mortality rates increased to 10 times in "moderate" smokers (15-24 cigarettes/day) and to 21 times in "heavy" smokers (> 25 cigarettes/day) compared to non-smokers. Smoking therefore poses an enormous health threat compared to not smoking, but the number of cigarettes smoked also has important effects.

The possible harmful effects of passive smoking have received considerable attention [38]. Although exposure is small compared to active smokers, non-smoking individuals in the same room or house with smokers show pulmonary deposition of particles as well as increased blood levels of nicotine and carboxyhemoglobin [39]. Infants and children living in the same household as parents or siblings who smoke are especially vulnerable, the effect being greater with maternal than paternal smoking [40]. In infants exposed to passive cigarette smoke, normal lung growth and development may be affected. Because the horse race effect predicts that a decrease in expiratory flow at an early age may contribute to a more rapid subsequent decline in lung function, even small changes in "starting lung function" may be critical.

With the intent of lowering toxic and addictive effects of cigarette smoking, the tar and nicotine contents in cigarettes have been reduced from 43 mg and 2.8 mg, respectively, in 1955 to 15 mg and 1 mg, respectively, in 1980 [41]. However, tar content reduction does not necessarily imply an equivalent reduction in the amount of toxic components in tobacco smoke [32]. Furthermore, smokers may adapt to lighter cigarettes by smoking increased numbers or inhaling more deeply [32]. Data on more recent extremely light cigarettes are still relatively limited.

Atmospheric Air Pollution

Since the beginning of the twentieth century it has been recognised that heavily industrialised areas have occasionally witnessed dramatic increases in mortality clearly linked to high levels in air pollution. Among the most renowned episodes is the heavy London smog in December 1952 which resulted in approximately 4000 excess deaths, particularly among patients with respiratory diseases [42]. A similar episode occurred in Donora, in Pennsylvania in 1948, where excess deaths were attributed to inhalation of sulphur oxide and particulate material [43]. The effects of ambient air pollution, both outdoor and indoor, are now well recognised and available evidence conclusively demonstrates that COPD can be aggravated by pollution exposure with consequent effects on COPD exacerbations, hospital admissions, and mortality [44, 45].

Air pollution is the result of the accumulation of substances generated by man, to levels that may be harmful to health. Most pollutants are associated with combustion of fossil fuels by industrial plants, urban heating systems, and car engines.

Major air pollutants include reducing agents (mainly carbonaceous particulate matter and sulphur dioxide), and oxidising substances consisting of hydrocarbons, oxides of nitrogen, and pollutants of photochemical reactions (ozone, aldehydes). Two main categories of pollution have been identified:

1. Industrial smog, a combination of smoke and fog often found in cold, damp, heavily industrialised areas. Products of industrial fuel combustion are mainly sulphur oxide and particulate material;
2. Photochemical smog, the result of high density car engine emissions. It usually represents a problem in hot sunny climates, where photochemical reactions with nitrogen oxides, carbon monoxide, and ozone may be facilitated.

It is generally thought that the effects of air pollution are minor compared to the influence of cigarette smoking [46], and there is little evidence that urban air pollution can per se cause COPD in non-smokers [47]. However, a study conducted expressly to address this question suggested that residence in heavily polluted areas is associated with an excess decline in FEV_1 over and above that attributable to smoking and other potential risk factors [48]. In this study, the effect of heavy pollution was only slightly less than the effect attributed to heavy smoking. If these results should be confirmed, ambient pollution may be likely to exert a broadly similar order of magnitude effect as smoking in the development of COPD.

Occupational Pollution

Increased risk of COPD has been described in relation to a number of occupations, generally involving exposure to dust or fumes. These effects are related to coal dust [49], silica [50], cadmium [51], animal feeds [52], and other dust, fume or solvent exposure [53, 54]. These studies are fraught with potential pitfalls due to the possible coexistence of other more substantial risk factors (mainly cigarette smoking). A review of cross-sectional and longitudinal studies that have addressed occupational dust exposure revealed that in some occupations there is unequivocal evidence for a significant effect of dust on lung function [55]. Respiratory symptoms are certainly more common among subjects with occupational exposure to dusts, and a dose-response relationship has been identified between incidence of respiratory symptoms and years of exposure to dusts [56].

Infection

Among the factors traditionally considered to play a role in the natural history of COPD are respiratory infections [57]. Potentially, infections may affect patients in a number of ways: recurrent acute infectious exacerbations and chronic colonisation and/or infection may favour progressive loss in lung function; bacterial exacerbations may be directly involved in mortality associated with COPD; and early life respiratory infections may affect the propensity to develop COPD in adult life [58].

Although acute infection is widely recognised as capable of causing acute deterioration in respiratory function, the exact role in determining irreversible damage is still debated. Among major prospective studies assessing the natural history of COPD, a correlation between infection and loss of respiratory function was found by some but not by others [59, 60].

Further insight into the association between infection and COPD will be extensively reviewed in the following chapters.

COPD and Genetics

Despite the clear association between smoking and COPD, there remains marked interindividual variation in the response to cigarette smoke. It has been estimated that only 10%-20% of chronic heavy smokers will ever develop symptomatic COPD [61]. This suggests that genetic factors may interact with environmental exposure in the development of airway disease. Epidemiological and clinical data indicate familial clustering of COPD [62, 63], higher correlation between parents and children, or between siblings than between spouses [64], and decreased prevalence of the disease with increased genetic distance [65]. Studies in monozygotic twins indicate that susceptibility to cigarette smoke in one twin predicts loss of lung function in both twins, whereas non-susceptible twins concomitantly maintain normal lung function in spite of cigarette smoking [66, 67]. No such evidence was recorded in dizygotic twins. Identification of genes involved in the susceptibility to COPD encounters the same difficulties arising with other complex diseases such as hypertension and diabetes mellitus, where a clear Mendellian pattern of inheritance is absent [68, 69].

Alpha$_1$-antitrypsin (α_1-AT) is a powerful antiprotease produced by the liver, blood monocytes and alveolar macrophages. Over 70 variants have been identified, among which the most common are identified as M, S, and Z [70]. Homozygous MM individuals express full proteolytic activity, whereas homozygous ZZ present severely impaired activity [71]. In these patients low levels of circulating α_1-AT are found and an accelerated decline in lung function occurs with onset of symptomatic COPD fairly early in life [72]. Homozygosity for this mutation is relatively rare in the general population but intermediate genotypes are more common. Evidence linking heterozygous α_1-AT genotypes and COPD is contradictory. Several population and longitudinal studies found associations between MZ genotype and increased prevalence of COPD, decreased lung function, and greater loss in elastic recoil compared to MM individuals [73-75]. However, others failed to confirm these findings in the general population [76, 77].

Alpha$_1$-antichymotrypsin (α_1-ACT) is similar to α_1-AT in that both are protease inhibitors. Two point mutations in the α_1-ACT gene have been identified and associated with decreased α_1-ACT serum concentrations and COPD [78, 79].

Homozygous deficiency or defective function of the cystic fibrosis transmembrane regulator (CFTR) gene regulating chloride movement across airway epithelial cell wall results in cystic fibrosis. Approximately 600 variants of the CFTR gene have been identified, the most common mutation being ΔF508 [80]. Although heterozygosity for this mutation is apparently associated with disseminated bronchiectasis, its role in the development of COPD is unsupported [81]. Other less common CFTR mutations have been associated with COPD in the absence of bronchiectasis in some patients [82], a finding not confirmed by other authors [83, 84].

Vitamin D-binding protein (VDBP), in addition to its role in vitamin metabolism, has been shown to influence the intensity of inflammatory reactions by enhancing the chemotactic activity of complement factors towards neutrophils, and acting as a macrophage-activating factor [85, 86]. Common isoforms of VDBP have been termed 1F, 1S and 2. COPD patients apparently show a greater likelihood for a homozygote 1F genotype, whereas genotypes containing the 2 allele (2-1F, 2-1S, and particularly 2-2) present a protective effect [87]. This association remains controversial and has not been replicated [88].

The blood group ABO antigens are secreted into saliva, plasma and respiratory secretions in approximately 80% of the population. It has been shown that nonsecretors have greater loss in lung function compared to secretors [89]. Similarly, Lewis blood group secretory status has been found to affect susceptibility to airflow obstruction [90]. Blood group factors may participate in adhesion of bacterial agents thus increasing susceptibility to infection.

Hereditary immunoglobulin A (IgA) and immunoglobulin G (IgG) deficiencies, alone or in combination, are known to favour recurrent infections. Both deficiencies have been evaluated in association with the development of COPD. A significant correlation between IgG2 levels and FEV_1 values was found in one study [91], whereas a selective IgA deficiency was found to segregate with COPD in a large family pedigree [92].

Other candidate genes for increased susceptibility to COPD include alpha$_2$-microglobulin [93], human leukocyte antigen (HLA) class I genes [88], cytochrome P4501A1 [94], extracellular superoxide dismutase [95], haptoglobin [96], and cathespin G [97]. Proof linking particular genotypes and COPD for the above genes is uncertain at best.

The basic derangement in COPD is a decrease in expiratory airflow. Different pathophysiological processes may contribute to development of the disease, including smooth muscle hypertrophy, inflammatory narrowing of peripheral airways and loss of elastic recoil [98]. Susceptibility to these processes may be linked to differing genetic bases that may contribute to a different extent in certain individuals.

Natural History

Lung function, expressed as FEV_1 values, increases from birth during childhood and peaks in early adulthood (approximately at the age of 20 years) [99]. This age may vary among different populations and according to sex. Maximal growth is followed by a "plateau phase", roughly between 25-35 years of age, during which variations in lung function are minimal [100]. After the age of 40 years, lung function starts to decline as a part of the age-related decrease in lung elastic recoil, slightly earlier in females than in males [100]. Reduced lung function levels in adult life may be a cause of reduced childhood growth, premature start of decline, or accelerated decline, in any combination. It has been recognised that lung function (adjusted for age and body weight) remains remarkably constant over time in non-smokers. The clinical implication is that lung function level in 10-20 years can be predicted from current values with a high degree of certainty (the "tracking" effect) [101].

The concept that susceptibility to COPD may be estimated by defining models of decline of pulmonary function was first introduced by Fletcher, et al. [33]. This study suggested that FEV_1 declines at a rate of approximately 36 ml/year in non-smoker males aged 30-59 years. This rate increases to approximately 44-55 ml/year in smokers. However, a subgroup of "susceptible" smokers may develop losses twice as evident (up to 70-120 ml/year). These data were subsequently confirmed by another group [100]. The rate of decline in lung function with age in non-smokers may cause a fall in FEV_1 of approximately 1 litre over 50 years. In most smokers the rate of decline is greater than in non-smokers, though often asymptomatic. In the subgroup of susceptible heavy smokers, lung function declines at a much higher rate than in average smokers and lung function can fall below 2 l. These subjects often present symptoms, mainly dyspnoea on exertion. Symptoms related to airflow limitation generally progress with further loss of lung function. Severe limitation of physical performance commonly occurs when FEV_1 values decline below 1 litre [6, 102].

Therefore, although approximately 50% of smokers develop symptoms of chronic bronchitis, only 10%-20% of susceptible heavy smokers go on to develop progressive airway obstruction [61]. This observation has led to intensive research in the natural history of COPD. Two important hypotheses which have influenced research are known as the "Dutch" and the "British" hypotheses. In broad terms the former emphasises the role of hypersensitivity in modulating airway response to irritant exposure, whereas the latter underscores the role of infections and irritants.

The British Hypothesis

The British hypothesis is based on the identification of airway irritants and infection as major factors influencing COPD natural history. It has been suggested that a variety of inhaled irritants may cause simple bronchitis. The ensuing mucus hyperproduction would then lead to airway obstruction and increased susceptibility towards infection. Long-term airway infections would bring about inflammatory derangements in the airways and lung tissues causing destruction and scarring. This in turns leads to permanent airflow obstruction. The theory was initially put forward in Great Britain in a period when industrial air pollution and cigarette smoking showed a steep rise, and when chronic bronchitis and COPD were emerging as important public health menaces. Fletcher, et al. [33] noted a significant association between loss of lung function and mucus hyperproduction, although this association was lost in a multivariate analysis. Furthermore, no association was found between mucus hypersecretion and COPD mortality [34]. Airway obstruction and mucus hypersecretion were therefore regarded as independent manifestations of the effects of cigarette smoking, and mucus hypersecretion considered an "innocent spectator", its presence not being invaluable for the development of invalidating airway obstruction [33]. The British hypothesis subsequently lost popularity, although a French 1980s study questioned the role of hypersecretion as an "innocent disorder" [103], associating mucus production with COPD mortality, and a recent study suggested that mucus hypersecretion may be related to FEV_1 even when corrected for confounding factors [104].

The Dutch Hypothesis

In the 1970s, a group of Dutch investigators proposed a hypothesis for the selective development of COPD observed in some smokers [105]. Termed the "Dutch hypothesis" [106], it states that patients with an atopic tendency and increased non-specific bronchial hyperresponsiveness (NSBH) have a higher risk for developing irreversible airflow obstruction. In individuals with hyperresponsive airways, repeated episodes of acute bronchoconstriction related to smoke inhalation may possibly cause airway remodelling and fixed airway narrowing. Alternatively, an exaggerated inflammatory response to smoke in atopic individuals may represent the basis of this association. The association between NSBH and airway function was then confirmed by other cross-sectional studies [107, 108], and high peripheral eosinophil blood counts and skin test positivity were also linked to respiratory symptoms [109].

Unlike asthmatic subjects, in whom NSBH may occur in the presence of normal baseline measurements of lung function, NSBH in COPD is associated with abnormal "prechallenge" lung function. Since initial FEV_1 is a known risk factor for the development of COPD, it was suggested that the relationship between NSBH and decline in FEV_1 could be spurious [106]. Later longitudinal studies provided further proof that increased rates of decline in FEV_1 are observed in hyperresponsive subjects, independent of smoking study [110, 111]. The reported excess decline in FEV_1 reached up to 25.6 ml/year in responders [110].

As not all smokers develop airway obstruction, Fletcher, et al. [33] postulated that there is a susceptible group of smokers. It was suggested that the presence of hyperresponsiveness may identify the susceptible smoker [112], although others suggested that hyperresponsiveness is the result of abnormal geometry following prolonged smoking and resulting in increased susceptibility to "real life stimuli" [113].

Is There an "American Hypothesis"?

The Dutch and the British hypotheses have generally been regarded as competing theories. However both are supported by reliable data and may rather be
considered as complementary. An initiating factor, as for example cigarette
smoking, leads to airway inflammation. In the Dutch hypothesis, this inflammatory process may lead to airway hyperreactivity. In the British hypothesis, it can
lead to infection and mucus hypersecretion, eventually contributing to fixed
airflow limitation. Rennard [102] suggested the existence of a third possibility,
that the inflammatory process directly leads to airway remodelling and airflow
limitation independently of airway hyperresponsiveness or mucus hypersecretion. This is probably obtained by upsetting the balance between tissue damage
and the mechanisms for tissue repair.

Conclusions

COPD is a heterogeneous collection of conditions that can affect various struc-
tures within the lung in different ways. These various processes can all result in
limitation of expiratory airflow. If severe enough, COPD will be present. The
various conditions that can lead to this syndrome are prevalent and often
relentlessly progressive. Although the disease comes to expression during late
adult life, early life events may be of great importance, both because of accumulation of risks and because of the strong tracking of pulmonary function.

A less favourable track for lung function development may start during
pregnancy. Risk factors include maternal smoking, poor nutrition, allergens,
and genetic predisposition. Risk factors during lung function growth include
poor lung function at birth, passive and active smoking, poor nutrition, air pollution, bronchial hyperresponsiveness, skin test positivity, eosinophilia, and
poverty. During the plateau phase risk factors include submaximal lung growth,
active smoking, hyperresponsiveness, air pollution, poor nutrition and poverty.
Lung function decline is accelerated by smoking, bronchial hyperresponsiveness, occupational exposure, poverty, and nutritional factors.

References

1. Ciba Guest Symposium (1959) Terminology, definitions, and classification of
   chronic pulmonary emphysema and related conditions. Thorax 14:286-299
2. American Thoracic Society (1962) Statement by the Committee on Diagnostic
   Standards for Nontuberculous Respiratory Diseases: Definitions and classification
   of chronic bronchitis, asthma, and pulmonary emphysema. Am Rev Respir Dis
   85:762-768
3. Fletcher CM, Pride NB (1984) Editorial: Definitions of emphysema, chronic bronchitis, asthma, and airflow obstruction: 25 years on from the CIBA symposium.
   Thorax 39:81

4. Canadian Thoracic Society Workshop Group (1992) Guidelines for the assessment and management of chronic obstructive pulmonary disease. Can Med Assoc J 147:420-424

5. Siafakas NM, Vermeire P, Pride NB, et al., on behalf of the Task Force (1995) ERS Consensus Statement. Optimal assessment and management of chronic obstructive pulmonary disease (COPD). Eur Respir J 8:1393-1420

6. American Thoracic Society (1995) Standards for the diagnosis and care of patients with chronic obstructive pulmonary diseases. Am J Respir Crit Care Med 152:878-883

7. The COPD Guidelines Group of the Standards of Care Committee of the BTS (1997) BTS guidelines for the management of chronic obstructive pulmonary disease. Thorax 52:S1-S28

8. Dow L, Coggon D, Osmond C, Holgate ST (1991) A population survey of respiratory symptoms in the elderly. Eur Respir J 4:267-272

9. Boezen M, Schouten JP, Postma DS, Rijcken B (1995) The relation between respiratory symptoms, pulmonary function and peak flow variability in adults. Thorax 50:121-126

10. Singh GK, Matthews TJ, Clarke SC, et al. (1994) Annual summary of births, marriages, divorces, and deaths: United States 1994. National Center for Health Statistics, Hyattsville (Monthly vital statistics report, vol. 43, n. 13)

11. – (1994) Morbidity and mortality chartbook on cardiovascular, lung, and blood diseases. National Heart, Lung and Blood Institute, Bethesda

12. – (1998) Strategies in preserving lung health and preventing COPD and associated diseases. The National Lung Health Education Program (NLHEP). Chest 113(2):123S-163S

13. Oswald NC (1959) Chronic bronchitis and emphysema: A symposium II. Clinical aspects of chronic bronchitis. Br J Radiol 32:289-292

14. Fletcher CM (1959) Chronic bronchitis. Its prevalence, nature, and pathogenesis. Am Rev Respir Dis 80:483

15. World Health Organization (1975) International classification of disease, 9th revision. WHO, Geneva

16. Benson V, Marano MA (1994) Current estimates from the National Health Interview Survey, 1993. National Center for Health Statistics, Washington (Vital and health statistics 10(190), DHHS publication no. (PHS) 95-1518)

17. Wilder C (1973) Prevalence of selected chronic respiratory conditions: United States, 1970. National Center for Health Statistics, Washington (Vital and health statistics 10(84), DHEW publication no. (HRA) 95-1518)

18. Tirimana PR, van Schayack CP, den Otter JJ, et al. (1996) Prevalence of asthma and COPD in 1992: has it changed since 1977? Br J Gen Pract 46:277-281

19. Collins JC (1993) Prevalence of selected chronic respiratory conditions: United States, 1986-1988. National Center for Health Statistics, Washington (Vital and health statistics 10(182), DHHS publication no. (PHS) 93-1510 415

20. Feinleib M, Rosenberg HM, Cillons JG, et al. (1989) Trends in COPD morbidity and mortality in the United States. Am Rev Respir Dis 140:S9-S18

21. Lung and Asthma Information Agency (1992) Trends in asthma mortality in the elderly. 92:1

22. Thom TJ (1989) International comparisons in COPD mortality. Am Rev Respir Dis 140(Suppl):S27-S34

23. Higgins MW, Thom TJ (1989) Incidence, prevalence and mortality: Intra- and intercountry differences. In: Hensley MJ, Sauders NA (eds) Clinical epidemiology of chronic obstructive pulmonary disease. Marcel Dekker, New York, pp 23-43

24. Davis RM, Novotny TE (1989) Changes in risk factors. The epidemiology of cigarette smoking and its impact on chronic obstructive pulmonary disease. Am Rev Respir Dis 140(Suppl):S82-S84

25. Higgins MW (1989) Chronic airways disease in the United States. Trends and determinants. Chest 96(Suppl):328S-334S
26. Miller GJ (1974) Cigarette smoking and irreversible airways obstruction in the West Indies. Thorax 29:495-504
27. Cullen KJ, Stenhouse NS, Welborn TA, et al. (1968) Chronic respiratory disease in a rural community. Lancet 2:657-660
28. Lange P, Groth S, Nynoe J, et al. (1990) Decline of the lung function related to the type of tobacco smoked and inhalation. Thorax 45:22-26
29. Beck GJ, Doyle CA, Schacter EN (1981) Smoking and lung function. Am Rev Respir Dis 123:149-155
30. Harris JE (1983) Cigarette smoking among successive birth cohorts of men and women in the United States during 1900-1980. J Natl Cancer Inst 71:473-479
31. United States Public Health Service (1964) Smoking and health. Report of the Advisory Committee of the Surgeon General. U.S. Government Printing Office, Washington 44:277. (PHS publ. 1103)
32. United States Public Health Service (1964) The health consequences of smoking. Chronic obstructive lung disease: A report of the Advisory Committee of the Surgeon General. U.S. Government Printing Office, Rockville, 9, 75-118, 185-260, 348-352, 361-412. (DHHS publ. (PHS) 84-50205)
33. Fletcher C, Peto R, Tinker C, Speizer FE (1976) The natural history of chronic bronchitis and emphysema. Oxford University, Oxford
34. Peto R, Speizer FE, Cochrane AL, et al. (1983) The relevance in adults of air-flow obstruction, but not of mucus hypersecretion, to mortality from chronic lung disease. Am Rev Respir Dis 128:491-500
35. Xu X, Weiss ST, Rijcken B, Schouten JP (1994) Smoking, changes in smoking habits, and rate of decline in FEV1: new insight into gender differences. Eur Respir J 7:1056-1061
36. Burchfield CM, Marcus EB, Curb JD, et al. (1995) Effects of smoking and smoking cessation on longitudinal decline in pulmonary function. Am J Respir Crit Care Med 151:1778-1785
37. Doll R, Peto R, Wheatley K, et al. (1994) Mortality in relation to smoking: 40 years' observation on male British doctors. BMJ 309:901-911
38. Leuenberger P, Schwartz J, Ackermannliebrich U, et al. (1994) Passive smoking exposure in adults and chronic respiratory symptoms (SALPALDIA study). Am J Respir Crit Care Med 150:1222-1228
39. Jarvis MJ, Russell MAH, Feyerabend C (1983) Absorption of nicotine and carbon monoxide from passive smoking under natural conditions of exposure. Thorax 31:829-833
40. Burchfiel CM, Higgins MW, Keller JB, et al. (1986) Passive smoking in childhood. Respiratory conditions and pulmonary function in Tecumseh, Michigan. Am Rev Respir Dis 133:966-973
41. United States Public Health Service (1979) Smoking and health. A report of the Surgeon General. U.S. Government Printing Office, Washington 4:1-7; 5:1-74; 6:1-52 8:1-93. (DHEW publ. PHS 79-50066)
42. Logan WPD (1953) Mortality in London fog incident. Lancet 1:336-338
43. Shrenk HH, Heimann H, Clayton GD, et al. (1949) Air pollution in Donora, PA: Epidemiology of the unusual smog episode of October 1948. Preliminary report. Public Health Service, Washington (Public health bulletin 306)
44. Bascom R, Bromberg PA, Costa DA, et al. (1996) Health effects of outdoor air pollution. Am J Crit Care Med 153:3-50

45. Lebowitz MD (1996) Epidemiological studies of the respiratory effects of air pollution. Eur Respir J 9:1029-1054

46. Morgan WKC (1986) On dust, disability and death (editorial). Am Rev Respir Dis 134:639

47. Zapletal A, Jech J, Paul T, et al. (1973) Pulmonary function studies in children living in an air-polluted area. Am Rev Respir Dis 107:400-409

48. Tashkin DP, Detels R, Simmons M, et al. (1994) The UCLA population studies of chronic respiratory disease. 6. Impact of air pollution and smoking on annual change in forced expiratory volume in one second. Am J Crit Care Med 149:1209-1217

49. Attfield MD, Hodous TK (1992) Pulmonary function of US coal miners related to dust exposure estimates. Am Rev Respir Dis 145:605-609

50. Hnizdo E (1992) Loss of lung function associated with exposure to silica dust and with smoking and its relation to disability and mortality in South Africa gold miners. Br J Ind Med 49:472-494

51. Davidson AG, Newman Taylor AJ, Darbyshire J, et al. (1988) Cadmium fume inhalation and emphysema. Lancet 1:663-667

52. Smid T, Heederik D, Houba R, Quanjer PH (1992) Dust and endotoxin-related respiratory effects in the animal feed industry. Am Rev Respir Dis 146:1474-1479

53. Nejjari C, Tessier JF, Dartigues JF, et al. (1993) The relationship between dyspnoea and main lifetime occupation in the elderly. Int J Epidemiol 22:848-854

54. Bakke PS, Baste V, Hanoa R, Gulsvik A (1991) Prevalence of obstructive lung disease in a general population: relation to occupational title and exposure to some airborne agents. Thorax 6:863-870

55. Becklake MR (1989) Occupational exposures: evidence for a causal association with chronic obstructive pulmonary disease. Am Rev Respir Dis 140(Suppl):S85-S91

56. Korn RJ, Dockery DW, Speizer FE, et al. (1987) Occupational exposures and chronic respiratory symptoms. A population-base study. Am Rev Respir Dis 136:298-304

57. Wilson R (1998) The role of infection in COPD. Chest 113:242S-248S

58. Murphy TF, Sethi S (1992) Bacterial infection in chronic obstructive pulmonary disease. Am Rev Respir Dis 146:1067-1083

59. Fletcher C, Peto R (1977) The natural history of chronic airflow obstruction. Br Med J 1:1645-1648

60. Kanner RE, Renzetti AD Jr, Klauber MR, Smith CB, Golden CA (1979) Variables associated with changes in spirometry in patients with obstructive lung diseases. Am J Med 67:44-50

61. Bascom R (1991) Differential susceptibility to tobacco smoke: possible mechanisms. Pharmacogenetics 1:102-106

62. Madison R, Zelman R, Mittman C (1980) Inherited risk factors for chronic lung disease. Chest 77(2 Suppl):255-257

63. Tager IB, Rosner B, Tishler PV, Speizer FE, Kass EH (1976) Household aggregation of pulmonary function and chronic bronchitis. Am Rev Respir Dis 114:485-492

64. Devor EJ, Crawford MH (1984) Family resemblance for normal pulmonary function. Ann Human Biol 11:439-448

65. Redline S, Tishler PV, Rosner B, et al. (1989) Genotypic and phenotypic similarities in pulmonary function among family members of adult monozygotic and dizygotic twins. Am J Epidemiol 129:827-836

66. Webster PM, Lorimer EG, Man SFP, Woolf CR, Zamel N (1979) Pulmonary function in identical twins: comparison of nonsmokers and smokers. Am Rev Respir Dis 119:223-228

67. Hankins D, Drage C, Zamel N, Kronenberg R (1982) Pulmonary function in identical twins raised apart. Am Rev Respir Dis 125:119-121

68. Soubrier F, Lathrop GM (1995) The genetic basis of hypertension. Curr Opin Nephrol Hyperten 4:177-181
69. Davies JL, Kawaguchi Y, Bennett ST, et al. (1994) A genome-wide search for human type 1 diabetes susceptibility genes. Nature 371:130-136
70. Cox DW, Johnson AM, Fagerhol MK (1980) Report of nomenclature meeting for alpha1-antitrypsin. Hum Genet 53:429-433
71. Janus AD, Philips NT, Carrell RW (1985) Smoking, lung function and alpha1-antitrypsin deficiency. Lancet 1(8421):152-154
72. Brantley ML, Paul LD, Miller BH, et al. (1988) Clinical features and history of the destructive lung disease associated with alpha1-antitrypsin deficiency of adults with respiratory symptoms. Am Rev Respir Dis 138:327-336
73. Klayton R, Fallat R, Cohen AB (1975) Determinants of chronic obstructive pulmonary disease in patients with intermediate levels of alpha1-antitrypsin. Am Rev Respir Dis 112:71-75
74. Tattersall SF, Pereira RP, Hunter D, et al. (1979) Lung distensibility and airway function in intermediate alpha1-antitrypsin deficiency. Thorax 34:637-646
75. Tárjan E, Magyar P, Váczi Z, et al. (1994) Longitudinal lung function study in heterozygous PiMZ phenotype subjects. Eur Respir J 7:2199-2204
76. Morse JO, Ldebowitz MD, Knudson RJ, Burrows B (1977) Relation of protease inhibitor phenotypes to obstructive lung diseases in a community. N Engl J Med 296:1190-1194
77. Bruce RM, Cohen BH, Diamond EL, et al. (1984) Collaborative study to assess the risk of lung disease in Pi Mz phenotype subjects. Am Rev Respir Dis 130:386-390
78. Poller W, Faber J-B, Scholz S, et al. (1992) Mis-sense mutation of α1-antichymotrypsin gene associated with chronic lung disease. Lancet 339:1538
79. Poller W, Faber J-B, Weidinger S, et al. (1993) A leucine-to-proline substitution causes a defective α1-antichymotrypsin allele associated with familial obstructive lung disease. Genomics 17:740-743
80. Kerem B-S, Rommens JM, Buchanan JA, et al. (1989) Identification of the cystic fibrosis gene: genetic analysis. Science 245:1073-1080
81. Gervais R, Lafitte J-J, Dumur V, et al. (1993) Sweat chloride and ΔF508 mutation in chronic bronchitis or bronchiectasis. Lancet 342:997
82. Pignatti PF, Bombieri C, Marigo C, et al. (1995) Increased incidence of cystic fibrosis gene mutations in adults with disseminated bronchiectasis. Hum Mol Genet 4:635-636
83. Gasparini P, Savoia A, Luisetti M, et al. (1990) The cystic fibrosis gene is not likely to be involved in chronic obstructive pulmonary disease. Am J Respir Cell Mol Biol 2:297-299
84. Artlich A, Boysen A, Bunge S, et al. (1995) Common CFTR mutations are not likely to predispose to chronic bronchitis in Northern Germany. Hum Genet 95:226-228
85. Kew RR, Webster RO (1988) Gc-globulin (vitamin D-binding protein) enhances the neutrophil chemotactic activity of C5a and C5a des Arg. J Clin Invest 82:364-369
86. Yamamoto N, Homma S (1991) Vitamin D-binding protein (group-specific component) is a precursor for the macrophage-activating signal factor for lysophosphatidylcholine-treated lymphocytes. Proc Natl Acad Sci USA 88:8539-8543
87. Horne SL, Cockcroft DW, Dosman JA (1990) Possible protective effect against chronic obstructive airways disease by the GC 2 allele. Hum Hered 40:173-176
88. Kaufmann F, Kleisbauer J-P, Cambon-de-Mouzon A, et al. (1983) Genetic markers in chronic airflow limitation: a genetic epidemiology study. Am Rev Respir Dis 127:263-269
89. Haines AP, Imeson JD, Meade TW (1982) ABH secretor status and pulmonary function. Am J Epidemiol 115:367-370

90. Horne SL, Cockroft DW, Lovegrove A, Dosman JA (1985) ABO, Lewis and secretor status and relative incidence of airflow obstruction. Dis Markers 3:55-62
91. O'Keefe S, Gzel A, Drury R, et al. (1991) Immunoglobulin G subclasses and spirometry in patients with chronic obstructive pulmonary disease. Eur Respir J 4:932-938
92. Webb Dr, Condemi JJ (1974) Selective immunoglobulin A deficiency and chronic obstructive lung disease. Ann Intern Med 80:618-621
93. Poller W, Barth J, Voss B (1989) Detection of an alteration of the alpha2-microglobulin gene in a patient with chronic lung disease and serum alpha2-microglobulin deficiency. Hum Genet 83:93-96
94. Cantlay AM, Lamb D, Gillooly M, et al. (1995) Association between CYP1A1 gene polymorphism and susceptibility to emphysema and lung cancer. J Clin Pathol Mol Pathol 48:M210-214
95. Peno-Green L, Crapo JD, Folz RJ (1995) Characterisation of human serum extracellular superoxide dismutase variants in normal and lung disease individuals. Am J Respir Crit Care Med 151:A167
96. Abe T, Kobayashi N, Yoshimura K, et al. (1991) Expression of the secretory leukoprotease inhibitor gene in epithelial cells. J Clin Invest 87:2207-2215
97. Lüdecke B, Poller W, Olek K, Bartholomé K (1993) Sequence variant of the human cathepsin G gene. Hum Genet 91:83-84
98. Sandford AJ, Weir TD, Paré PD (1997) Genetic risk factors for chronic obstructive pulmonary disease. Eur Respir J 10:1380-1391
99. Burrows B, Cline MG, Knudson RJ, et al. (1983) A descriptive analysis of the growth and decline of the FVC and FEV1. Chest 83:717-724
100. Sherill DL, Camilli A, Lebowitz MD (1989) On the temporal relationship between lung function and somatic growth. Am Rev Respir Dis 140:638-644
101. Dockery DW, Berkey CS, Ware JH, et al. (1983) Distribution of forced vital capacity and forced expiratory volume in one second in children 6-11 years of age. Am Rev Respir Dis 128:405-412
102. Rennard SI (1998) COPD: Overview of definitions, epidemiology, and factors influencing its development. Chest 113:235S-241S
103. Annesi I, Kaufmann F (1986) Is respiratory mucus hypersecretion really an innocent disorder? Am Rev Respir Dis 134:688-693
104. Vestbo J, Prescott E, Lange P (1996) Association of chronic mucus hypersecretion with FEV1 decline and chronic obstructive pulmonary disease morbidity. Am J Crit Care Med 153:1530-1535
105. Van der Lende R, Visser BF, Wever-Hess J, et al. (1973) Distribution of histamine threshold values in a random population. Reveu de l'Institut d'Hygiene des Mines Hasselt (Belgium) 28:186-190
106. Weiss ST, Speizer FE (1984) Increased level of airways responsiveness as a risk factor for development of chronic obstructive lung disease: what are the issues? Chest 86:3
107. Sparrow D, O'Connor G, Colton TH, et al. (1987) The relationship of nonspecific bronchial responsiveness to the occurrence of respiratory symptoms and decreased levels of pulmonary function. Am Rev Respir Dis 135:1255-1260
108. Rijcken B, Schouten JP, Weiss ST, et al. (1988) The relationship between airway responsiveness to histamine and pulmonary function level in a random population sample. Am Rev Respir Dis 137:826-832
109. Mensinga TT, Schouten JP, Rijcken B, et al. (1990) The relationship of eosinophilia and positive skin test reactivity to respiratory symptom prevalence in a community-based population study. J Allergy Clin Immunol 86:99-107
110. Villar MT, Dow L, Coggon D, et al. (1995) The influence of increased bronchial responsiveness, atopy and serum IgE on decline in FEV1; a longitudinal study in the elderly. Am J Respir Crit Care Med 151:656-662

111. Rijcken B, Schouten JP, Xu X, et al. (1995) Airway hyperresponsiveness to histamine is associated with accelerated decline of FEV1. Am J Respir Crit Care Med 151:1377-1382
112. Pride NB (1988) Bronchial hyperactivity in smokers. Eur Respir J 1:485-487
113. Burrows B, Martinez FD (1989) Bronchial responsiveness, atopy, smoking and chronic obstructive pulmonary disease (editorial). Am Rev Respir Dis 140:1515-1517

Acute Exacerbations of Chronic Bronchitis: In Search of a Definition

P. BALL

Introduction

"They [exacerbations] are extremely difficult to grade and undoubtedly some patients do want to please a doctor who has shown more than usual interest in their tiresome and commonplace disease" [1].

"The value of future work ... would be increased if agreement could be reached on the definition of an exacerbation" [2].

These sentiments regarding chronic bronchitis, expressed 30 years ago, illustrate a disease which has received relatively slight attention over the years, despite its enormous economic and healthcare implications. Regrettably, most pulmonologists and microbiologists have found other facets of the interface between the infectious process and structural lung disease more interesting. This indifference is reflected in the attitudes of many family practitioners – for example in the low priority given to acute exacerbations of chronic bronchitis (AECB) in terms of hospital admission compared with pneumonia [3]. Despite the consensus on a primary definition of the disease [4, 5], there remains little consistency in the criteria under which patients are admitted to trials of therapy for its exacerbations. Thus meaningful analyses and meta-analyses of data from differing studies and centres are frequently invalidated.

Thus, at the close of the millennium, at a time when antibiotics with enormously increased potency and respiratory tissue penetration have become available, clinical investigation frequently fails to demonstrate improved results when these drugs are compared with existing therapy. As a result, few data are available which enable rational choices of therapy.

This may in part be due to mismatching of trial entry criteria, confusion as to the relative importance of risk factors in severity classifications, reliance on traditional short-term outcome measures and failure to define additional out-

School of Biomedical Sciences, University of St. Andrews, Fife, Scotland

comes by which true differences can be demonstrated. For all of these aspects definitions are of paramount importance. However, for such a heterogeneous disease [6, 7], it is sensible to review the current position before attempting to offer solutions.

Early Development of Definitions

The first mention in the medical literature of an inflammatory disease of the airways described as chronic bronchitis (CB) and associated with excessive mucus production appears to have been in the early nineteenth century [8]. Distinctions between chronic bronchitis and other causes of chronic obstructive pulmonary disease (COPD) were delayed a century further. Wall in 1907 [9] clearly noted underlying causes, such as spasmodic asthma or tuberculosis of the lungs, as separate entities, described recurrent acute attacks – termed exacerbations, made lifestyle recommendations, including a suggestion of "migration to a warmer climate" (French or Italian Riviera) and propounded principles of management. The latter, of course, made no mention of antibacterial chemotherapy, although vaccines "prepared from organisms isolated from the sputum" were considered to have produced satisfactory results. The disease was clearly recognisable as a distinct syndrome, but then as now more by exclusion than design.

Fifty years later, Oswald, et al. [10] reiterated the diagnostic triad of cough, sputum and breathlessness and emphasised the heterogeneity of the affected population. The predominance of middle aged and elderly males common to later surveys [6, 11] was established and the roles of environmental pollution and tobacco smoking were defined. In over 1000 patients, 88% had spasmodic and 52% constant breathlessness. Some 85% gave histories indicating exacerbations, sputum volume almost always increasing at that time and becoming purulent in two-thirds. About 15% of patients had constant purulent sputum in both winter and summer, and 95% of males were smokers [10].

A pattern had thus emerged which, although based on clinical observation and exclusion of other, better-defined diseases, allowed recognition of a separate entity.

However, the statements which precede this discussion reflect a situation, where, 25 years into the chemotherapeutic era, there was little consensus either as to the nature and precipitations of COPD exacerbations or indeed the role of respiratory pathogens in both the acute phase and in the longer term deterioration of airway function. Neither was there a clear view of the role, if any, that antibacterial chemotherapy might play. It is pertinent to consider whether, after a further 25 years, much has changed.

The Current Disease

In the US, the mortality rate for chronic obstructive pulmonary disease (COPD) due primarily to cigarette smoking has increased dramatically since the 1970s, at a time when all other causes of death have been in decline [12, 13]. Ninety percent of patients with COPD suffer from chronic bronchitis [12]. COPD, the fourth-leading cause of death in North America, probably affects more than 15 million Americans [14]. It is responsible for more than 100 000 deaths and 500 000 admissions to hospital annually [15]. At the turn of the decade in the UK, the cost of antibiotic therapy alone for this disease approached £50 million and an excess of 25 000 000 working days were lost each year [16]. Despite the apparent continuity of CB and asthma as causes of COPD, the two are usually readily distinguished by general practitioners [6]. A recent study in family practice found accurate differentiation of asthma from COPD to be possible using a simple formula. This incorporated three symptoms - wheeze, dyspnoea and allergen-induced symptoms – plus gender and pack-years of smoking [17].

The major risk factors for COPD are tobacco smoking [18], a family history of obstructive lung disease, exposure to atmospheric, domestic and occupational pollutants, and recurrent respiratory tract infections, particularly during infancy [19]. However other contributing factors may not be immediately apparent from the northern hemisphere. Thus, in developing countries, probably more than 50% of cases in women of lower socio-economic status and many in men are caused by exposure to biomass fuel smoke (usually wood, straw or crop residue smoke) in cooking and light industry [20, 21].

The availability of such statistics clearly implies that reporting doctors have little difficulty in recognising the disease and, indeed, worldwide the disease presents a remarkably and consistently similar pattern, an average of 5%-7% of the adult male population being affected [22]. However, the failure of primary antibiotic therapy in 13%-25% of cases [6, 23] indicates that, whereas diagnosis may not be at issue, severity rating and appropriate therapy clearly is.

Definitions in the Era of Chemotherapy

A number of learned societies and consensus groups have proposed disease definitions that betray similar roots and incorporate fundamental misassumptions by which features of an established exacerbation are taken to indicate degree of severity. In fact, most of the clinical features so utilised are present between exacerbations. Thus, the European Respiratory Society (ERS) consensus statement [5] characterises COPD by reduced maximum expiratory flow unchanged over several months and defines chronic bronchitis by the presence of chronic or recurrent increase in bronchial secretions sufficient to cause cough. These secretions are present on most days for a minimum of 3 months in two successive years and are not attributable to other cardiac or pulmonary causes. Airflow obstruction is not an essential criterion. A large scale survey in the UK confirmed that most practitioners used precisely these criteria plus increases in sputum and dyspnoea to define an exacerbation [6].

The ERS definition itself derives from that of the American Thoracic Society (ATS) [4]. The UK Medical Research Council [24], whilst acknowledging the ATS view, chose more pragmatically to classify the disease into 3 groups:
- Simple chronic bronchitis,
- Chronic or recurrent muco-purulent chronic bronchitis, and
- Chronic obstructive bronchitis.

The essential diagnostic criterion was bronchial hypersecretion, although bacterial infection was also recognised frequently to occur.

Others have used functional classifications, based on relationships between increasing mortality and decreasing FEV_1 [14], which correlate with the types of pathogen causing the infective exacerbation [25]. However, in contrast to pneumonia [26] such classifications have not been validated in terms of outcome.

The Infectious Diseases Society of America (IDSA) Guidelines for Evaluation of new anti-infective drugs [27] require ATS / ERS basic criteria plus "some (*undefined*) combination of increased cough, dyspnoea, sputum volume or purulence". Italian studies have attempted to integrate such features into a scoring system to establish severity [28] and both Latin American and Asia Pacific Consensus Groups [29, 30] have produced Guidelines for Management. These use a severity classification based on ATS / ERS criteria plus the presence or absence of certain risk factors, considered to predicate poor outcome of standard chemotherapy. However, the introduction to the ERS's latest (1998) guidelines for adult community-acquired lower respiratory tract infections (LRTI) states that "attempts to identify the type of LRTI ... are probably unhelpful outside hospital" [31]. In the opinion of this reviewer, that is a retrograde step. The overwhelming reason to define chronic bronchitis and AECB in the community is to enable appropriate specific management principles to be applied to the relevant patients to prevent complications, early recurrence and hospital admission.

Defining the Effect of Treatment

Consistent amongst these definitions and classifications is the premise that antibiotics have value in acute exacerbations of chronic bronchitis. In acute bronchitis there is general agreement that their value is limited [32], although two recent meta-analyses have shown either a trend in favour [33] or evidence of modest benefit [34]. Similar failures of individual antibiotic studies in AECB to show significant differences either compared to placebo or between themselves have distorted appreciation of the role of chemotherapy.

In contrast to studies of other diseases, e.g. urinary tract infections or community-acquired pneumonia, which compare treatments or active therapy to placebo, those in AECB have rarely used consistent inclusion criteria. Many have included patients with asthma, pneumonia and acute bronchitis in a heterogeneous melee from which little reliable information could or did emerge. Thus, the few placebo-controlled studies of antibiotics during the 1960s to mid-1980s gave conflicting results.

More positive evidence awaited the landmark "Winnipeg" [35] and the equally important but less often quoted Italian study by Allegra and co-workers [28]. These large scale surveys not only established the efficacy of antibiotic therapy in defined exacerbations, later confirmed by a meta-analysis of all trials [36], but also firmly secured the basic criteria for an exacerbation requiring antibiotic treatment. Thus Winnipeg type 1 exacerbations [35] and those with significant scores based on the Italian system [28] have increased dyspnoea, sputum production and sputum purulence (in addition to cough and in many cases small airway obstruction). These features are the cardinal criteria of an exacerbation.

However, the Winnipeg classification into three groups (for the purposes of excluding insignificant, often viral exacerbations) is often misinterpreted. Type 1 exacerbations which fulfil all the cardinal criteria are commonly but erro-neously believed to be of greater severity – notably by pharmaceutical compa-nies who promote products for such patients by variously describing them as "sick, ill or requiring special attention". In fact, few studies based on Winnipeg type 1 criteria alone show the new, more active and kinetically improved com-pounds to have any advantages over existing antibiotics. This is unsurprising: such advantages are unlikely to become apparent in patient groups for whom the spontaneous placebo responses exceed 80% [37, 38]. Even studies which showed better responses (after tetracycline compared with placebo) did so only in patients with "moderately severe" attacks [39].

The Canadian and Italian studies define a true exacerbation but, in turn, demand the development of a severity classification based on risk factors for poor outcome. By such means, clinical response and the potentially greater effi-cacy of improved, compared with standard antibiotics can be assessed. To achieve this purpose, it is necessary to establish predictive risk factors.

Studies Defining Risk Factors for Poor Outcome

A large scale survey of UK general practice in the early 1990s assessed 471 patients with AECB to determine the relationship of disease pattern to treat-ment outcome [6]. The following patient characteristics were noted:
- Mean duration of disease was 12 years.
- 82% were current or ex-smokers.
- 100% of patients had cough and produced sputum every day.
- 100% were breathless.
- 45% were moderately to severely breathless during the exacerbation.
- 57.5% of patients had moderate or severe airflow obstruction.
- 37.4% of patients had < 3 exacerbations in the previous year.
- 30.8% of patients had 3-4 chest exacerbations in the previous year.
- 31.8% of patients had > 4 exacerbations in the previous year.
- 38.0% of patients suffered co-existent cardiopulmonary disease.

The cardinal symptoms of chronic bronchitis, dyspnoea and increased sputum volume and purulence – the Winnipeg type 1 criteria [35] – were present in almost every case, but did not predict treatment failure. Thus, the definition of an exacerbation was confirmed but a link to severity and thus to outcome was absent. However, poor therapeutic outcome was predicted to a high degree of statistical significance by either the presence of co-existent cardiopulmonary disease, 4 or more exacerbations in the previous 12 months, or both [6]. These factors, together with decreasing FEV_1, are known to exert a negative influence on the exacerbation-free interval [40]. In addition, mucus hypersecretion has been confirmed to correlate with death from pulmonary infection, defining not only a risk factor but a further piece in the jigsaw of causality and mortality [41, 42].

To these factors a number of existing risk predictors from the literature can be added, most of which are clearly associated with severe disease of long standing. These include:
- Development of acute respiratory failure [43],
- Advancing age and delay in intensive care unit (ICU) referral [44],
- Continued smoking between exacerbations [45],
- Frequent requirements for domiciliary steroid therapy [46].

A further large-scale, domiciliary study in Canada [11] has subsequently shown that prolonged duration of disease (>10 years) and advancing age also predicted poor treatment outcomes. It further demonstrated that patients with multiple risk factors responded better to an antibiotic with improved potency and respiratory tissue penetration (ciprofloxacin) than to standard drugs. In fact 15% of individuals studied had 5 risk factors and almost 50% had two or more. These studies allow definitions of severity to be proposed and subsequently tested in clinical populations.

Outcomes

Criteria for objective assessment of therapy outcome have been suggested [7] and include:
- Overall response assessment (clinical and microbiological)
- Microbiological assessment of sputum 1 week after cessation of therapy
- Speed of recovery of individual symptoms
- Time until the next infective exacerbation
- Requirement for subsequent therapy within defined periods.

To these, certain additional and desirable parameters might be added, including pharmaco-economic analyses and quality of life assessments. Pharmaco-economic studies are not yet required by registration authorities but are increasingly demanded by managed care organisations making decisions regarding formulary inclusion. Quality of life (QoL) assessment [47] requires scoring systems, such as the St. George's Respiratory Questionnaire (SGRQ) [48]. These have been validated in related diseases, for example, in bronchiectasis [49]. Similar systems deserve attention in AECB in which, for example, time and rate of return to the pre-exacerbation state might differentiate antibiotic classes. SGRQ assessments have been used to show that, although physiological measurement may change little in AECB, other major changes in subjective health status may take many weeks to return to baseline [50]. Indeed, such assessments can measure significant treatment-related improvements in QoL despite less impressive changes in respiratory function [47, 51].

Bacterial Eradication and Clinical Failure

Definitions of disease and severity enable comparisons of treatment regimes, outcomes and their costs to the individual and to society. There may be considerable cost-benefit from improved outcomes after primary therapy. A retrospective review of the literature since 1990 [52] found a high correlation (r = 0.90) between failure to eradicate causative bacteria and clinical failure. A study in Germany showed that hospitalisation following clinical failure of first-line therapy is the key cost driver in out-patients with more severe pneumonia and AECB [53]. In the UK, the excess cost occasioned by hospitalisation following treatment failure may far outweigh primary care costs [54], again suggesting that effective therapy targeted against defined patient groups might significantly reduce overall cost burdens.

Conversely, drug performance can be comparatively assessed by measuring the exacerbation-free interval following therapy of AECB [55], prolongation of which implies fewer exacerbations and complications (including hospitalisations) in the following year. Both ampicillin (for sensitive organisms) and fluoroquinolones perform well in this respect. Most recently, Chodosh and colleagues [56, 57] compared ciprofloxacin with both cefuroxime axetil and clarithromycin, all administered for 14 days. Initial clinical response was identical (93% vs. 90% and 90% vs. 82%, respectively, in evaluable patients). Bacterial eradication with ciprofloxacin was better than with either cefuroxime axetil (96% vs. 82%, $p < 0.01$) or clarithromycin (91% vs. 77%, $p = 0.01$). However, in contrast to earlier findings with oral cephalosporins such as cefaclor [55], there was no difference in infection-free interval after cefuroxime (178 days) and ciprofloxacin (146 days; $p = 0.37$), nor after clarithromycin (51 days) and ciprofloxacin (142 days; $p = 0.15$), despite the apparent trend in the latter comparison.

Debate surrounds the undoubted differences between antibiotic classes in relation to exacerbation-free interval. For example, how can antibiotics maintain influence weeks after their elimination, especially when it is recognised that even the most effective fail completely to eradicate *H. influenzae* [58]. Other factors are known to influence this interval, notably pre-existing consultation patterns and satisfaction [59], degree of FEV_1 impairment, co-morbidity and number of previous exacerbations [40]. Definitions of response should include at least discussion of such parameters.

The Future

In view of the conclusions reached by various authors and learned bodies over the last decade, it is to be hoped that international agreement can now be reached on the following.

First, chronic bronchitis can be defined as a *chronic* disease characterised by mucus hypersecretion causing cough and sputum to be present for at least 2-3 months in every year over the previous 3 years [4, 24], subject to exacerbations. The latter, for the purposes of clinical trial entry, should be characterised by all three cardinal criteria: increased breathlessness, increased sputum volume, and sputum purulence [35].

Second, risk factors predictive of poor response to standard therapy can be identified, including:
- Advanced aged [11]
- Prolonged history (> 10 years) [11]
- Continued tobacco smoking [45]
- 4 or more exacerbations within the previous 12 month [6]
- Significant cardiopulmonary co-morbidity [6]
- Mucus hypersecretion [42]
- Previous requirements for corticosteroid therapy, use of domiciliary oxygen, and superimposed episodes of acute respiratory failure

Third, a simple classification can be used to identify patients in whom various forms of antimicrobial therapy are indicated. A suggested classification would comprise the following stages of disease:
- *Stage I: simple bronchitis.* Acute bronchitis, usually viral, in patients with no underlying airway disease plus early chronic disease not fulfilling the 3-year time constraint imposed by the ATS classification, in which antibiotic therapy would rarely be required [32].
- *Stage II: simple chronic bronchitis* fulfilling the ATS definition, but lacking risk factors for poor outcome. Antibiotic therapy for patients with such mild disease might comprise short-course treatment with basic agents, e.g. oral broad-spectrum penicillins, subject to local resistance prevalence amongst *H. influenzae, M. catarrhalis* and *S. pneumoniae.*
- *Stage III: complicated chronic bronchitis* defined as for Stage II but also characterised by the presence of at least one risk factor for poor outcome. Patients in this group would require antibiotics proven to have (a) high potency and low resistance prevalence against the major pathogens and (b) high concentrations in bronchial mucosa and surrounding parenchymal lung tissue (> serum concentrations). Whenever possible, these agents should have shown proven benefit in meta-analyses of randomised clinical trials (RCT) or at least one large-scale, double-blind RCT in comparison to standard therapy and, preferably, also to placebo. Unless based on such Category Ia / Ib evidence, guidelines might have little influence on prescribing patterns [60].
- *Stage IV: chronic bronchial sepsis* comprising a group with severe airways disease, frequently shown to have bronchiectasis and commonly chronically infected with enteric gram-negative bacilli plus *P. aeruginosa* [25].

Such proposals have enabled the promulgation and wide-spread acceptance of supra-national, severity classification-based guidelines in both Latin America [29] and the Asia-Pacific region [30].

Finally, these criteria should be adopted as entry standards for clinical trials. Trials in patients classified as Stage III might finally allow us to prove that drugs which are better kinetically and in vitro are actually better for our most at-risk patients. As recently stated, "Patients enrolled into clinical studies should satisfy criteria to ensure that the disease is of sufficient severity to detect differences in efficacy between treatments" [7]. Without such constraints clinical assessments of valuable compounds will remain incapable of revealing their true potential because of inadequate trial design. Real progress will not be made in this field until conformity of practice in definition and severity assessment is established.

References

1. Petersen ES, Esmann V, Honcke P, et al. (1967) A continuing study of the effect of treatment on chronic bronchitis. Acta Med Scand 182:293-305
2. Fisher M, Akhtar AJ, Calder MA, et al. (1969) Pilot study of the factors associated with exacerbations in chronic bronchitis. Br Med J 4:187-192
3. Schaberg T, Gialdroni-Grassi G, Huchon G, Leophote P, Manresa F, Woodhead M (1996) An analysis of decisions by European general practitioners to admit to hospital patients with lower respiratory tract infections. Chest 51:1017-1022
4. American Thoracic Society (1962) Chronic bronchitis and asthma, and pulmonary emphysema. A statement by the Committee on Diagnostic Standards for Non-tuberculous Respiratory Diseases. Am Rev Respir Dis 85:762-768
5. Siafakis NM, et al. (1995) ERS consensus statement: Optimal assessment and management of chronic obstructive pulmonary disease (COPD). Eur Resp J 8:1398-1420
6. Ball P, Harris JM, Lowson D, Tillotson G, Wilson R (1995) Acute infective exacerbations of chronic bronchitis. Q J Med 88:61-68
7. Wilson R, Tillotson G, Ball P (1996) Clinical studies in chronic bronchitis: a need for better definition and classification of severity. J Antimicrob Chemother 37:205-208
8. Badham C (1808) Observations on the inflammatory affections of the mucous membranes of the bronchiae. London
9. Wall C (1907) Bronchitis, chronic. In: Hutchinson R (ed) Index of treatment. Wright and Sons Bristol, Simkin Marshall, London, 12th edn 1940, pp 110-113
10. Oswald NC, Harold JT, Martin WJ (1953) Clinical pattern of chronic bronchitis. Lancet 2:639-643
11. Grossman R, Mukherjee J, Vaughan D and the Canadian Ciprofloxacin Health Economic Study Group (1998) A 1-year community-based health economic study of ciprofloxacin vs. usual antibiotic treatment in acute exacerbations of chronic bronchitis. Chest 113:131-141
12. Higgins MW, Thorn T (1990) Incidence, prevalence and mortality: Intra- and inter-country differences. In: Hensley MJ, Saunders NA (eds) Clinical epidemiology of chronic obstructive pulmonary disease. Marcel Dekker, New York, pp 23-43
13. Higgins M (1993) Epidemiology of pulmonary disease. In: Casaburi R, Petty TL (eds) Principles and practice of pulmonary rehabilitation. WB Saunders, Philadelphia, pp 10-17

14. American Thoracic Society (1995) Standards for the diagnosis and care of patients with chronic obstructive pulmonary disease. Am Rev Respir Dis 152:S78-S83

15. – (1996) Morbidity and mortality: 1996 chartbook on cardiovascular, lung and blood Diseases. National Heart, Lung, and Blood Institute, National Institutes of Health, Bethesda, p 52

16. Ball P, Tillotson G, Wilson R (1995) Chemotherapy for chronic bronchitis: controversies. Presse Med 24:189-194

17. Thiadens HA, De Bock GH, Dekker FW, et al. (1998) Identifying asthma and chronic obstructive pulmonary disease in patients with persistent cough presenting to general pratictioners; descriptive study. Brit Med J 316:1286-1290

18. Wynder EL, Fairchild EP Jr (1996) The role of a history of persistent cough in the epidemiology of lung cancer. Am Rev Respir Dis 94:709-720

19. Sherrill DL, Lebowitz MD, Burrows B (1990) Epidemiology of chronic obstructive pulmonary disease. Clin Chest Med 11:375-387

20. Smith KR, Aggarwal AL, Dave RM (1983) Air pollution and rural biomass fuel in developing countries: a pilot study in India and implications for research and policy. Atmos Environ 17:2343-2362

21. Dennis RJ, Maldonado D, Norman S, Baena E, Martinez G (1996) Woodsmoke exposure and risk for obstructive airways disease among women. Chest 109:115-119

22. Ball P, Make B (1998) Acute exacerbations of chronic bronchitis: an international comparison. Chest 113(Suppl):199S-204S

23. MacFarlane JT, Colville A, Guion A, MacFarlane RM, Rose DH (1993) Prospective study of aetiology and outcome of adult lower respiratory tract infections in the community. Lancet 341:511-514

24. – (1965) Report to the Medical Research Council. Definition and classification of chronic bronchitis for clinical and epidemiological purposes. Lancet 1:775-779

25. Eller J, Ede A, Schaberg T, Niederman MS, Mauch H, Lode H (1998) Infective exacerbations of chronic bronchitis: relation between bacteriologic etiology and lung function. Chest 113:1542-1548

26. Fine MJ, Auble TE, Yealy DM, Hanusa BH, Weissfeld LA, Sinder DE, et al. (1997) A prediction rule to identify low-risk patients with community acquired pneumonia. N Engl J Med 336:243-250

27. Chow AW, Hall CB, Klein JO, et al. (1992) Evaluation of new anti-infective drugs for the treatment of respiratory tract infections. Clin Infect Dis 15(Suppl 1):S62-S88

28. Allegra L, Grassi C, Grossi E, Pozzi E, Blasi F, Frigerio D, Nastri A (1991) Ruolo degli antibiotici nel trattamento delle riacutizza della bronchite cronica. Ital J Chest Dis 45:38-48

29. Jardim JR and the Latin American Consensus Group (1997) Consenso Latinamericano sobre infecciones en bronquitis cronica. Revista Panamericana de Infectilogia 1:3-19

30. Balgos AA and the Consensus Group (1988) Guidelines for the role of antibiotics in acute exacerbations of chronic bronchitis in the Asia Pacific region: report and recommendations of a consensus group. Med Prog 25:29-38

31. Huchon G, Woodhead M, Gialdroni-Grassi G, et al. (1998) Guidelines for management of adult community-acquired lower respiratory tract infections. Eur Respir J 11:986-991

32. Orr PH, Scherer K, MacDonald A, Moffat MEK (1993) Randomised placebo-controlled trials of antibiotics for acute bronchitis: a critical review of the literature. J Fam Pract 36:507-512

33. Fahey T, Stocks N, Thomas T (1998) Quantitative systematic review of randomised controlled trials comparing antibiotic with placebo for acute cough in adults. BMJ 316:906-910

34. Becker L, Grazier R, McIsaac,W, Smucny J (1999) Antibiotics for acute bronchitis (Cochrane Review). Update Software, Oxford (Cochrane Collaboration, Cochrane Library, issue 1)

35. Anthonisen NR, Manfreda J, Warren CPW, Hershfield ES, Harding GKM, Nelson NA (1987) Antibiotic therapy in exacerbations of chronic obstructive pulmonary disease. Ann Intern Med 106:196-204

36. Saint S, Bent S, Vittinghof E, Grady D (1995) Antibiotics in chronic obstructive pulmonary disease exacerbations: a meta-analysis. JAMA 273:957-960

37. Elmes PC, King TC, Langlands JHM, et al. (1965) Value of ampicillin in the hospital treatment of exacerbations of chronic bronchitis. Br Med J 2:904-908

38. Nicotra MB, Rivera M, Awe RJ (1982) Antibiotic therapy of acute exacerbations of chronic bronchitis: a controlled study using tetracycline. Ann Intern Med 97:18-21

39. Berry DG, Fry J, Hindley EJ, et al. (1960) Exacerbations of chronic bronchitis: treatment with oxytetracycline. Lancet 1:237-139

40. Miravitlles M, Mayordomo C, Artes MT and the EOLO group (1997) Factors influencing the exacerbation-free time in COPD: results of follow-up of the EOLO study. Eur Respir J 10(Suppl 25):148S

41. Lange P, Nyboe J, Appleyard M, Jensen G, Schnor P (1990) The relation of ventilatory impairment and of chronic mucus hypersecretion to mortality from obstructive lung disease and from all causes. Thorax 45:579-585

42. Prescott E, Lange P, Vestbo J (1995) Chronic mucus hypersecretion in COPD and death from pulmonary infection. Eur Respir J 8:1333-1338

43. Derenne JP, Fleury B, Pariente R (1988) Acute respiratory failure of chronic obstructive lung disease. Am Rev Resp Dis 138:1006-1033

44. Seneff MG, Wagner DP, Wagner RP, et al. (1995) Hospital and 1-year survival of patients admitted to intensive care units with acute exacerbation of chronic obstructive lung disease. JAMA 274:1852-1857

45. Burrows B (1987) The course and prognosis of different forms of chronic airways obstruction in a sample from the general population. N Engl J Med 317:1309-1314

46. Strom K (1993) Survival of patients with chronic obstructive pulmonary disease receiving long-term domiciliary oxygen therapy. Am Rev Respir Dis 147:585-591

47. Donner CF, Carone M (1998) Determing quality of life in COPD patients. RT Int Fall:37-43

48. Jones PW, Quirk FH, Baveystock CM, Littlejohns P (1992) A self-complete measure of health status for chronic airflow limitation: the St. George's Respiratory Questionnaire. Am Rev Respir Dis 145:1321-1327

49. Wilson CB, Jones PW, O'Leary CJ, Cole PJ, Wilson R (1997) Validation of the St. George's Respiratory Questionnaire in bronchiectasis. Am J Respir Crit Care Med 156:536-541

50. Anie K, Lowton K, Jones PW (1997) Changes in health status following an acute exacerbation of chronic bronchitis. Eur Respir J 10(Suppl 25):148S

51. Jones PW, Bosh TK (1997) Quality of life changes in COPD patients treated with salmetorol. Am J Respir Crit Care Med 155:1283-1289

52. Pechere J-C (1998) Modelling and predicting clinical outcomes of antibiotic therapy. Infect Med 15(Suppl E):46-54

53. Vogel F (1998) Cost benefits from improving clinical outcome. Infect Med 15 (Suppl E):61-67

54. McGuire A (1998) Burden and cost of LRTI: a methodologic overview. Infect Med 15(Suppl E):26-31

55. Chodosh S (1991) Treatment of acute exacerbations of chronic bronchitis: state of the art. Am J Med 91(Suppl 6A):87S-92S

56. Chodosh S, Schreurs A, Siami G and the Bronchitis Study Group (1998) Randomised, double blind study of ciprofloxacin and cefuroxime axetil for treatment of acute bacterial exacerbations of chronic bronchitis. Clin Infect Dis 27:722-729

57. Chodosh S, Schreurs A, Siami G and the Bronchitis Study Group (1998) Efficacy of oral ciprofloxacin vs. clarithromycin for treatment of acute bacterial exacerbations of chronic bronchitis. Clin Infect Dis 27:730-738

58. Groeneveld KL, van Alphen L, Eijk PP, et al. (1990) Endogenous and exogenous reinfections by *Haemophilus influenzae* in patients with chronic obstructive pulmonary disease; the effects of antibiotic treatment upon persistence. J Infect Dis 161:512–517

59. MacFarlane J, Holmes W, MacFarlane R, Britten N (1997) Influence of patients' expectations on antibiotic management of acute lower respiratory tract illness in general practice: questionnaire study. BMJ 315:1211-1214

60. Shekelle PG, Woolf SH, Eccles M, Grimshaw J (1999) Developing guidelines. BMJ 318:593-596

Acute Exacerbations of COPD: Methods and Role of Microbiology

S. Chodosh

Introduction

Diagnosis of an acute exacerbation of chronic obstructive pulmonary disease (AE/COPD) provides little guidance as to the appropriate therapy for the individual patient presenting with this syndrome. The problem is that the clinical presentation characteristic of acute exacerbation is not distinctive for a specific etiology. In addition, any single patient with COPD may have chronic bronchitis (CB), chronic bronchial asthma (CBA), pulmonary emphysema (CPE), or a combination of these upon which the AE is superimposed. Faced with this dilemma, many clinicians prefer to use COPD and avoid making the specific diagnoses. The occurrence of an AE in this setting now requires another "best guess" as to specific etiology, or to treat to cover the more common etiologies for the AE. The proper assessment of acute exacerbations is not assisted by using COPD as a description of the underlying bronchopulmonary disease. COPD is not a disease with a defined pathologic basis, but rather is a description of a physiologic abnormality common to many pathophysiologically different diseases. Although the three predominant diseases under COPD often co-exist in individual patients, specific therapeutic treatment for the individual patient depends on defining the role each play in the individual patient. A specific diagnosis is particularly important to the patient who only has CB, or CBA, or CPE. Despite the increasing knowledge of the important pathophysiologic differences in bronchial receptors and the inflammatory processes between CB and CBA, the shotgun approach to treatment at the clinical level remains popular. The airway obstruction that is due to emphysematous changes is not responsive to the majority of therapeutic modalities for CB and CBA. The severity of obstruction is defined by the degree and location of structural change secondary to the parenchymal damage characteristic of this disease.

The increase of bronchopulmonary symptoms and signs that characterize AE/COPD can be related to a number of different factors. The importance of identifying the specific causal factors for an AE is to provide guidance for the

Pulmonary Research Laboratory, Department of Veterans Affairs Outpatient Clinic, Boston, MA 02114, USA specific immediate therapy needed, as well as for planning preventive measures to avoid future recurrences. The majority of AE can be attributed to bacterial infection, viral infection, increased inhalation of toxic particles and gases, secretion clearance problems, decreases of background therapy, allergens, or structural changes of bronchopulmonary architecture. The latter etiology would be more common in patients with CPE relating to increases of the size of emphysematous bullae or a pneumothorax. Allergens as a stimulus for an AE are virtually only seen in patients with CBA. All of the other factors could be causes of AE in patients with CB, CBA, or both. Surprisingly, there are no prospective data on the incidence of these various etiologies of AE in COPD. Anecdotal references suggest that approximately 50% are due to bacterial infection with the rest related to other etiologies.

Diagnosis of Chronic Bronchopulmonary Diseases

Although not essential, defining which of the chronic bronchopulmonary diseases the patient has facilitates the evaluation and treatment of individual AE. Diagnosis of CB, CBA and CPE based on clinical symptoms and signs is not very precise. Chronic productive cough for at least 3 months of the year for 2 successive years are the clinical criteria for CB, but CBA in older patients often presents with the same symptoms. Wheezing and dyspnea are complaints common to all three diseases. Asthma as described in children and young adults is characterized by acute episodes of wheezing dyspnea with or without cough or sputum production. It is often seasonal or associated with specific allergens or physical triggers. In chronic bronchial asthma, the symptoms are present most of the time and cough and sputum are more prominent symptoms. The co-existence of both CB and CBA is not uncommon, with the onset of the CBA often occurring later in life – often when the patient with CB stops smoking. These patients may not have a history of childhood asthma or atopy. Based on clinical signs and symptoms, it is not surprising that lumping these clinically similar presentations under COPD has been so popular. Physical examination is also not very specific for any of the three main diseases. A layman can suspect the diagnosis of CPE based on the barrel chest, pursed-lip breathing and dyspnea, and the chest examination demonstrating hypersonance with low, fixed diaphragms tends to confirm this. However, most COPD patients with emphysema are not this overt. Rhonchi, course rales, diminished breath sounds, prolonged expiration and wheezing are also not differential.

The usual laboratory tests commonly available to the clinician only provide minimally useful data for a differential diagnosis. Blood eosinophilia is support for a diagnosis of CBA, but lack of this finding does not exclude the diagnosis. Elevation of blood IgE is also a variable finding in CBA. Radiologic chest procedures can define the presence and extent of CPE, with computed tomography more sensitive than a routine chest roentgenogram. Spirometry is useful for defining the degree of obstruction present, but not in determining the patho-physiologic basis for the obstruction. The differential response to beta-adrener-gic and anticholinergic bronchodilators also is not distinctive with considerable overlap of response between diseases. Many CB patients respond to beta-adren-ergic agents, and at least a third of CBA patients respond to anticholinergic challenge.

The most direct approach to differentiating CB and CBA has been known for over 100 years, but it has not been commonly employed in recent decades. A large number of investigations were compiled by von Hoesslin in 1926 [1], describing the nature of the inflammatory and epithelial cells in sputum char-acteristic of various diseases of the lung. This old "wheel" was reinvented in 1961 [2] and the characteristics of CB and CBA were quantitatively described in 1970-1972 [3-6]. The old and newer investigations reaffirmed that finding a pre-dominance of eosinophils in sputum was typical of asthma, while a predomi-nance of neutrophils was characteristic of CB and of other nonallergic bron-chopulmonary diseases. It has also been noted that treatment directed at a specif-ic etiology of sputum neutrophilia, e.g. bacterial infection, resulted in a marked reduction of sputum neutrophils. Inhalation of toxic smoke, e.g. as in smoke inhalation, results in a marked increase of sputum neutrophils [7]. In an analo-gous way, treatment of asthma with corticosteroids results in a marked decrease of sputum eosinophils, but does not affect the neutrophils in the bronchitic patient [8, 9]. The characteristics of the inflammatory response can be quickly and easily noted by examining an aliquot of whole, wet sputum microscopically [10, 11]. The pathophysiology of emphysema does not lead to sputum production. Therefore, the diagnosis of CPE depends on radiologic and physiologic criteria. Exacerbations of COPD are only rarely related to the emphysematous component of COPD.

The most efficient use of therapeutic agents for CB and/or CBA can be achieved when the diagnosis of one or both is known for the specific patient. This maximizes the long-term goals of management of these chronic diseases. This maxim is even more important when considering therapy for the AEs that occur in COPD. The inflammatory response to many of the causes of AE is usu-ally distinctive enough to direct the appropriate therapy for that acute event. Acute worsening of respiratory symptoms is common in COPD. Considering the large population base of patients with CB, CBA and/or CPE, the socioeco-nomic impact of these events is staggering. Despite this, the diagnosis and treatment of such episodes is often haphazard.

Determining the Etiology of Acute Exacerbations

Table 1 summarizes the differential value of the various diagnostic modalities available to the clinician for the reasonable identification of the differerent causes of AE occurring in chronic bronchial disease. Acute exacerbations of

Table 1. Acute exacerbations in chronic bronchial diseases: differential value of clinical and laboratory patterns for specific etiologies

Symptoms, signs and laboratory findings	Type of exacerbation					
	Bacterial	Viral	Irritant inhalation	Thickened secretions	Allergen-induced	Background therapy stopped
Bronchopulmonary symptoms & history	1[a]	1	3	2	2	4
Bronchopulmonary physical findings	0	0	0	0	0	0
Spirometry	0	0	0	0	0	1
Chest radiology	0	0	0	0	0	0
Routine lab tests						
Hematology	1	1	0	0	1	0
Chemistry	0	0	0	0	0	0
Urinalysis	0	0	0	0	0	0
Blood gases	0	0	0	0	0	0
Sputum cytology & gram stain	4	4	2	2	4	0
Gross characteristics	0	0	0	3	0	0
Bacteriology	2	0	0	0	0	0

[a] Differential value: *0*, none; *1*, minimally helpful; *2*, moderately helpful; *3*, fairly helpful; *4*, excellent

COPD of any etiology all present with similar increases of bronchopulmonary symptoms, although all may not be present. Most commonly those may include increases of cough frequency, cough severity, and sputum production with a change of the physical nature of the sputum to being thicker and more purulent. Other less frequent symptoms are increased dyspnea and/or wheezing, chest congestion, chest discomfort, and scant hemoptysis. Systemic symptoms of chilliness, feverishness, malaise or anorexia may also be present. However, shaking chills, fever or pleuritic pain usually suggest the presence of pneumonia. Physical examination may reveal as a new finding or as a worsening of rhonchi, coarse rales, wheezes, decreased breath sounds, prolongation of expiration, tachypnea and tachycardia. A minimally elevated body temperature may be noted. The above symptoms or signs are not diagnostic of any specific cause of the AE. A chest roentgenogram may occasionally reveal evidence of an infiltrate or atelectasis. Spirometry commonly demonstrates an increase of airways obstruction in all types of AE. The blood cell analysis may rarely show a mild leukocytosis with a left shift of neutrophils suggesting infection, or eosinophilia suggesting an allergic etiology.

There are no substantive data as to the incidence of the various etiologies of AE in COPD. The relative incidence likely varies dependent on local geographic and environmental conditions, as well as the time of the year. In the COPD patients with predominantly CB, it is estimated that 50% may be due to bacterial infection with the other portion divided among other etiologies. If CBA is the predominant factor in the COPD, then allergic causes would be more common. AE in CPE would be related to changes in emphysematous pathology and, consequently, are infrequent. The other etiologies of AE other than the common bacterial infection or allergen-triggered event include viral infection, increased inhalation of toxic gases and particles, difficulty in clearing secretions, decreases of background therapy or changes in environmental conditions or physical activity.

The circumstances in which the AE developed can provide clues as to the possible etiology. Viral infection is more likely when such infections are prevalent in the community or when close associates have similar symptoms. With viral infection, the systemic symptoms are often more prominent than in bacterial infection. The most common reason for AE due to increased inhalation of toxic gases and particles is an increase or renewal of cigarette smoking by the patient. COPD patients subjected to inhalation anesthesia or high air-pollution days will often have an increase of symptoms and signs. Difficulty in clearance of bronchial secretions commonly occurs when the home or work environment becomes excessively dry, such as with heating in cold weather. Acute increases of symptoms also are noted when patients stop their background supportive therapy. Exposure to cold, windy or very hot and humid days may lead to increased symptoms for patients with all types of COPD, as can an increase of physical activity. The importance of obtaining the circumstances under which the AE occurred is that the information can be used to correct the precipitating cause(s). This should lead to immediate benefit from specific therapy and also be useful in maintaining an improved clinical condition.

Sputum Evaluation

Determining the etiology of a specific exacerbation based solely on clinical and routine laboratory testing almost always results in a best-guess decision. The chosen therapy is usually based on what type of AE could hurt the patient most if not treated. The ability to establish the correct etiology of an AE in the classic COPD patient can be greatly enhanced by evaluation of the sputum produced as a result of the specific etiologic factors. Table 2 details the important differential characteristics available from sputum evaluation for the main types of AE. The nature of the inflammatory cell response, and the changes of the exfoliated bronchial epithelial cells and of the bacterial population provide key diagnostic

Table 2. Sputum characteristics of specific types of active exacerbations of chronic bronchitis with or without bronchial asthma

Sputum findings	Type of exacerbation					
	Bacterial	Viral	Irritant inhalation	Thickened secretions	Allergen-induced	Background therapy stopped
Volume	I	I	I	D	I	V
Cell concentration	I	I	I	I	I	V
Purulence	I	I	I	I	I	V
Neutrophils	I	I	I	NC	V	V
Eosinophils	D	D	D	NC	I	V
Bronchial epithelial cells	I	I[a]	I	NC	I[a]	V
Macrophages	V	NC	NC	NC	V	V
Bacteria on gram stain	I	NC	NC	NC	NC	NC

I, increased; D, decreased; V, variable change; NC, no change. [a] Swollen and in clusters

criteria for diagnosis. This type of examination does require the availability of a microscope, a few microscope glass slides and the capability to do a simple gram stain. It also requires training of patients in how to collect the necessary specimen with the least oropharyngeal contamination as possible. The value of sputum examination in evaluating AE in COPD is dismissed by many as being unreliable. However, such a conclusion is unwarranted if the three aspects of dealing with sputum are carefully followed: collection of the specimen over a time-period likely to contain material from the bronchopulmonary area, microscopic selection of an aliquot exclusive of oropharyngeal secretions, and utilization of this selected material for subsequent microscopic and cultural evaluations. Beside the value of such examination in the initial assessment of the AE, follow-up evaluations can monitor the response to treatment. Collection over a set time period insures that the specimen will contain material from whenever the patient clears secretion from the lung and provides a quantitative volume measure which reflects the extent and severity of the bronchopulmonary pathology. When the patient does not collect a specimen, a stat sample can also be useful. When a sample cannot easily be produced when being evaluated, obtaining one may be facilitated by chest percussion, postural drainage maneuvers or the use of inhaled aerosols to stimulate a productive cough. In very ill patients – usually in hospital – specimens may be obtained via tracheobronchial aspiration, bronchoscopy or trans-tracheal aspiration. Whatever the method for obtaining the specimen, it should always be assumed that some degree of oropharyngeal material will be mixed with that coming from the bronchopulmonary system.

Expectorated specimens invariably are a mixture of the pathologic material from the bronchopulmonary system (sputum) and secretions from the oropharynx. Selection of a sputum aliquot for examination can be facilitated by pouring the specimen into half of a petri dish [12]. Plugs or strands of denser material should be teased out, placed on a clean microscope slide and viewed under low power with reduced light. The presence of large oropharyngeal squamous cells indicates that the portion selected is not a satisfactory representation of the exudate produced in the damaged lung. Further evaluation of such specimens will not provide useful information. Finding macrophages in the specimen is a strong indicator that an appropriate aliquot has been selected. This aliquot should be used for the definitive examinations. A small part of this aliquot should be placed on another microscope slide and covered with a coverslip. This should be examined under high power to locate cellular areas and then evaluated using the oil immersion objective to identify the types of inflammatory and bronchial epithelial cells. An estimate of the percentage of neutrophils, eosinophils and macrophages can easily be determined. The nature of the pathologic change occurring in the bronchial epithelium can be assessed by observing if the exfoliated bronchial epithelial cells (BEC) are pyknotic, swollen or occurring individually or in clusters. In CB or in nonallergic causes of AE, the predominant inflammatory cell will be the neutrophil with less than 5% eosinophils and a variable number of macrophages. The BEC will be individual and pyknotic. The neutrophils will often demonstrate toxic granulations. In CBA, eosinophils will be over 10% and may be as high as 90%. These are often associated with the finding of Charcot-Leyden crystals, an eosinophil equivalent, particularly during recovery from an asthmatic AE. The BEC are swollen and clusters (creola bodies) are often noted. These simple observations of the sputum wet preparation provide immediate differentiation of allergic from nonallergic bronchial pathology.

Microbiological Evaluation

The specimen previously described should also be streaked on a microscope slide and gram stained. The numbers and morphologic types of bacteria present in good cellular areas free of any oropharyngeal squamous cells can be assessed. An increased number of bacteria associated with an increase of sputum neutrophils identifies bacterial infection as the cause of the AE. Table 2 shows the various distinctive patterns of inflammatory cells, BEC and bacterial elements which help define the nature of the various AE that commonly occur in COPD. The numbers of the commonly occurring bacterial pathogens in bacterial AE that constitute an increase have been defined [13]. These are more than 12 Haemophilus-like bacteria, 8 pneumococcal-like bacteria, 18 moraxella-like bacteria and/or 2 gram-negative bacilli. Wet preparations that are predominantly eosinophilic are unlikely to demonstrate increased numbers of bacteria on gram stain [14].

Microbiological identification of the specific pathogens responsible for the acute bacterial exacerbation is generally of little value in deciding appropriate therapy. Selection of an appropriate antimicrobial can be achieved based on the morphological identification of the organism on gram stain in the vast majority of cases. Therapy should not be delayed while waiting for the results of a culture or sensitivity tests. Exceptions to this are when organisms resembling staphylococci or gram-negative bacilli are seen on gram stain, when the initial treatment fails, or if the particular patient has been noted to carry resistant organisms in previous bacterial AE. However, the initial choice of antimicrobial should be one most likely to be effective against the 3 common pathogens, *Streptococcus pneumoniae*, *Haemophilus influenzae* and *Moraxella catarrhalis*, and with consideration for their increasing resistance to certain antimicrobials.

Conclusions

The differential diagnosis of the type of AE based on the clinical observations and the sputum examination should lead to the appropriate specific therapy of the acute episode. This approach is cost-effective and does not expose the patient to unnecessary risks of inappropriate therapy. Table 3 outlines in general the appropriate therapy for each type of AE. Although many of the therapeutic modalities are indicated for all of the types of AE, the primary or most important components should be stressed for the specific type of AE. It is perhaps just as important to know which treatments are not indicated for specific AEs. Utilization of the information available from sputum examination refines the approach to treatment and provides a more scientific basis to the art of clinical practice.

Table 3. Therapeutic considerations for acute exacerbations of chronic bronchitis with or without bronchial asthma

Therapy	Type of exacerbation					
	Bacterial	Viral	Irritant inhalation	Thickened secretions	Allergen-induced	Background therapy stopped
Antimicrobial	P	NI	NI	NI	NI	NI
Corticosteroid	NI	NI	NI	NI	P	NI
Hydration and inhalation	S	S	S	P	S	RAT
Avoidance of irritant inhalation	S	S	P	S	S	RAT
Expectorant	S	S	S	P	S	RAT
Bronchodilator	S	S	S	S	P	RAT

P, primary or most important therapy; *S*, secondary or supportive therapy; *NI*, not indicated; *RAT*, resume appropriate therapy

Note. The views expressed in this chapter are those of the author and do not reflect the official policy or position of the Department of Veterans Affairs of the United States Government.

References

1. Von Hoesslin H (1926) Das Sputum, Zweite Auflage. Verlag von Julius Springer, Berlin
2. Chodosh S, Zaccheo CW, Segal MS (1961) The cytology and histochemistry of sputum cells I. Preliminary differential counts in chronic bronchitis. Am Rev Respir Dis 85:635-648
3. Chodosh S (1970) Examination of sputum cells. N Engl J Med 282:854-857
4. Chodosh S, Medici TC (1971) The bronchial epithelium in chronic bronchitis I. Exfoliative cytology during stable, acute bacterial infection and recovery phases. Am Rev Respir Dis 104:888-898
5. Medici TC, Chodosh S (1972) Sputum cell dynamics in bacterial exacerbations of chronic bronchial disease. Arch Intern Med 129:597-603
6. Medici TC, Chodosh S (1972) The reticulo-endothelial system in chronic bronchitis I. Quantitative sputum cell populations during stable, acute bacterial infection and recovery phases. Am Rev Respir Dis 105:792-804
7. Faling LJ, Medici TC, Chodosh S (1974) Sputum cell population measurements in bronchial injury. Observations in acute smoke inhalation. Chest 65:565-595
8. Chodosh S (1978) Sputum: observations in status asthmaticus and therapeutic considerations. In: Weiss EB (ed) Status asthmaticus. University Park, Baltimore, pp 173-200
9. Baigelman W, Chodosh S, Pizzuto D, Cupples A (1983) Sputum and blood eosinophils during corticosteroid treatment of exacerbations of asthma. Am J Med 75:929-936
10. Chodosh S, Baigelman W, Pizzuto D (1975) Sputum, an approach for maximum clinical information. Am Family Physician 1975:116-121
11. Baigelman W, Chodosh S (1984) Sputum 'wet preps': window on the airways. J Respir Dis 5:59-70
12. Chodosh S (1977) Sputum cytology in chronic bronchial disease. Adv Asthma Allergy 4:8-27
13. Baigelman W, Chodosh S, Pizzuto D (1979) Quantitative sputum gram stains in chronic bronchial disease. Lung 156:265-270
14. Baigelman W, Chodosh S, Beiser A, Pizzuto D, Janowski R (1993) Sputum eosinophilia negates need to perform sputum gram's stain. Lung 171:15-18

Acute Exacerbations of COPD: Aetiology and Antibiotic Resistance

G. Nicoletti[1], R. Mattina[2], S. Stefani[1]

Introduction

The worldwide occurrence of acute exacerbations of chronic obstructive pulmonary disease (COPD), a persistent inflammation and irritation of the bronchial tree, is one of the most important problems which face researchers today. Patients who fall under the umbrella of the clinical definition of chronic bronchitis form a heterogeneous group due to the range of severity of the condition, its common association with airflow obstruction (which may or may not be reversible) and emphysema, and a variable susceptibility to infective exacerbations. Acute exacerbations of chronic bronchitis are common, but their cause may be difficult to identify and might include viral infections, environmental pollutants, allergic responses and bacterial infections. The cause may be multifactorial, so that viral infection or level of air pollution may exacerbate bronchitis, which in turn may predispose to secondary bacterial infections.

Bacteriological Diagnosis

Exacerbations of COPD are poorly understood in clinical terms and not easily defined in laboratory terms. Patients will often report a change in sputum colour, volume or viscosity accompanied by increased dyspnoea.

Cellular analysis of a fresh sputum specimen is necessary in the evaluation of every patient with chronic bronchitis. Continual bronchial irritation is indicated by the presence of many polymorphonuclear (PMN) granulocytes, even during the quiescent period of the disease. It is important to determine the number of eosinophils. Ciliated epithelial cells can be recognised, and their

[1] Department of Microbiological and Gynaecological Sciences, University of Catania, Catania, Italy; [2] Institute of Microbiology, University of Milan, Milan, Italy

number correlates reasonably well with the degree of vigorous coughing that was needed to produce the sputum specimen. Gram staining will often show a mixture of gram-positive and gram-negative bacteria that is consistent with contamination by normal mouth flora or with tracheal colonisation principally by *Haemophilus influenzae* and *Streptococcus pneumoniae* [1] as well as *Moraxella catarrhalis*.

The mucus secreted in chronic bronchitis contains various glycoproteins, mucopolysaccaride acids, and albumin. Small amounts of a number of immunoglobulin species are present including secretory IgA, IgG, occasionally IgM and IgE, or proteolytic fragments derived from them.

In severe exacerbations of chronic bronchitis, when hospitalisation is necessary, bacteriological diagnosis based on bronchoscopic samples is frequently indicated. These samples are obtained by bronchial washes or brushes, protected specimen brushing, bronchoalveolar lavage or transbronchial biopsy.

Relationship of Infection to Acute Exacerbations

The most enigmatic problem in chronic bronchitis is the role of bacterial infection. Although its exact place is uncertain, bacterial infection does not appear to initiate the disease. However, bacteria are probably significant in perpetuating the disease and may be critical in producing the characteristic exacerbations. Cultural methodologies currently used may not exclude oral flora that can contaminate sputum specimens. Pathogenic bacteria can be cultured from the bronchi in up to 82% of cases of chronic bronchitis. Routine sputum specimens from patients with chronic bronchitis commonly contain non-encapsulated *H. influenzae*, *S. pneumoniae*, and other oropharyngeal commensal flora, including *Moraxella catarrhalis* and *H. parainfluenzae*. In most cases, one or all of these species is recovered from approximately 70% of the sputum specimens and rightfully can be considered as the baseline microbial flora of many patients with chronic bronchitis.

The development of a purulent sputum is not correlated specifically with the presence of one or more of all these bacteria: however, evidence suggests that purulence is associated with a quantitative increase in the number of microorganisms cultured from sputum [2].

Recent epidemiologic studies have shown that in patients with acute respiratory tract infections, intracellular pathogens, and particularly *Mycoplasma pneumoniae* and *Chlamydia pneumoniae*, might be involved more frequently than was previously assumed [3]. Recent data of Blasi, et al. [4] demonstrated that at least 4% of exacerbations may be associated with *Chlamydia pneumoniae* infection.

Old and New Pathogens

The predominant organisms during acute infective exacerbations were believed to be *S. pneumoniae* and non-typable *H. influenzae*. Other microorganisms such as *Moraxella catarrhalis* and *H. parainfluenzae* were considered to be also involved [5-8]. Non-typable *H. influenzae* accounts for approximately 50%-70% of isolates from patients with acute exacerbations of chronic bronchitis, while *S. pneumoniae* is found with a lower frequency, between 10% and 20% [6, 7].

An active role of *H. influenzae* and *S. pneumoniae* was argued: it has been suggested that repeated or chronic bacterial infections initiate and perpetuate a cycle of airway damage based upon stimulation of inflammatory mechanisms by bacteria and their products [9].

In recent years, *H. parainfluenzae*, a microorganism which has never been considered a pathogen [10], has had an increasing frequency of isolation in COPD patients who undergo antibiotic treatment [6, 7, 11]. The more convincing evidence of its pathogenic role was the discovery that some strains of *H. parainfluenzae* can induce large amounts of histamine [12], contributing adverse effects. Continued monitoring of the results of sputum cultures shows a frequent isolation of *M. catarrhalis* in pure or in combined cultures, and infections sustained by this microorganism are now extensively described in many countries throughout the world [13], even if the factors responsible for this increase, such as changes in pathogenicity, are poorly understood. The natural habitat of *M. catarrhalis* is believed to be exclusively humans; the organism has been isolated from the nasopharynx and pharynx. Evidence of its direct pathogenic role in lower respiratory tract infections has been acquired [13-17].

The controversial results obtained on the contribution of these microorganisms to the pathogenesis of COPD, also due to the heterogeneity of patients included in the study, induced some researchers to hypothesise that in patients with advanced disease, gram-negative bacteria other than *Haemophilus* spp. play at least an equally important role [18]. The authors, hypothesising that these bacteria are partly involved in the progression of the disease, demonstrated that Enterobacteriaceae and *Pseudomonas* spp. are the predominant bacteria in patients with impaired respiratory functions (FEV$_1$) and hence are correlated with the severity of the disease. Another study has documented the correlation between *H. influenzae* and *P. aeruginosa* isolation with the greatest degree of functional impairment [19].

Finally, the association between *C. pneumoniae* and chronic bronchitis has been investigated, and it appears that approximately 5% of COPD acute exacerbations are sustained by this pathogen [4]. Recent data from the same group demonstrated that *C. pneumoniae* chronic infection may increase susceptibility to airway colonisation by other pathogens [20].

Asymptomatic Colonisation and Chronic Infection by *Haemophilus* spp.

Haemophilus influenzae and *H. parainfluenzae* live symbiotically in the upper respiratory tract of humans. With the occasional exception of the human genital tract, the human nasopharynx is the sole ecological niche occupied by these organisms; they are never found in the environment and do not colonise or infect other animal species. Nasopharyngeal colonisation by *H. influenzae*, which precedes *H. influenzae* infection and disease, is a dynamic process: colonisation begins early in life and may persist for prolonged periods of time also in the presence of *H. influenzae*-specific mucosal antibodies. Possible explanations for prolonged carriage include: (i) its known ability to persist intracellularly [21]; (ii) the induction of a weak inflammatory response by *H. influenzae* carriage [22]; and (iii) the presence of antigenic variations among colonising *H. influenzae* strains [23]. In addition to chronic, asymptomatic colonisation of healthy individuals, *H. influenzae* also chronically infects patients with underlying respiratory tract diseases: although these patients may be infected with one *H. influenzae* strain for a prolonged period of time, subtle changes in the surface antigens of the organisms result in new epitopes that are not recognised by antibodies specific for its original infecting strains [24]. Thus antigenic diversity, obtained by a number of unique biologic features and genetic mechanisms [25, 26], appears to be an important mechanism by which *H. influenzae* can avoid attack and can survive in the only environmental site that it normally occupies.

Bacterial pathogens isolated from sputum may persist in the lower airways of patients with severe disease between exacerbations. Groeneveld, et al. [25] in a three-year longitudinal study demonstrated that exacerbations in COPD coincide with endogenous or exogenous re-infection by *H. influenzae* biotype II, and antibiotic treatment was not effective in eradicating strains. Similar persistence and failure to eradicate infecting organisms has also been reported for *S. pneumoniae* in COPD [28].

Recent molecular data reported by Privitera, et al. [29] on unrelated isolates of *H. parainfluenzae* isolated from serial COPD patients (alone or as co-pathogens) show that isolates are genetically different, demonstrating re-infection with new strains and thus excluding persistence of infection or reinfection with a strain from the same lineage, except for two pairs of isolates. The strains, belonging to biotypes II and III, were subjected to phylogenetic analysis which demonstrated them to be heterogeneous and to spread among many genetically diverging lineages.

Resistance to Antibiotics

The emergence and spread of antibiotic resistance among human pathogens is certainly the most striking evolution that has arisen in bacteria within the past five decades. With only few exceptions, antibiotic resistance in bacterial pathogens was identified soon after the introduction of antibiotics into clinical practice, illustrating the genetic flexibility of bacteria.

The evolution of antibacterial resistance in human pathogenic and commensal microorganisms is the result of the interaction between antibiotic exposure and the transmission of resistance among microorganisms, but this also depends on the environment and the social habits of individuals. Among bacterial diseases, lower respiratory tract infections are a group of common diseases associated with a considerable burden, both for the patient and the healthcare system. The empiric management of community-acquired respiratory tract infections has been complicated by the emergence of high rates of antimicrobial resistance in respiratory pathogens such as *Streptococcus pneumoniae, Haemophilus influenzae, Haemophilus parainfluenzae,* and *Moraxella catarrhalis.* Although there are important geographical differences between countries and cities, this serious problem must be faced in different ways by continuous epidemiological surveillance and by performing studies on the molecular mechanisms of resistance at both the biochemical and genetic levels. It is vital that physicians make therapeutic choices based on this kind of information for bacterial eradication and clinical cure.

Surveillance Studies on Antibiotic Resistance: Comparison among Different National and International Studies

Nation-wide susceptibility surveillance studies have been performed all around the world to control the level of resistance of the main respiratory pathogens. Here we compare some international data with the Italian Epidemiological Observatory.

The Alexander Project is an ongoing, international multicentre study investigating antimicrobial susceptibility patterns in common respiratory pathogens [30], in both the United States and Europe. The incidence of beta-lactamase positive *H. influenzae* was 30.1% in the USA and 15.5% in Europe, and the incidence of beta-lactamase-positive *M. catarrhalis* has risen to > 90% in Europe and the United States (respectively, 92% and 96.5%).

The incidence of penicillin resistance in *S. pneumoniae* is higher in Europe (24.9%) than in the United States (12.3%); the geographical distribution of this resistance is very different in countries such as France and Spain where it is 40%. For the majority of centres included in the study, there is a marked association between penicillin and macrolide resistance in *S. pneumoniae,* with minimal inhibitory concentrations (MICs) for erythromycin > 32 mg/l in penicillin-resistant strains. Cross-resistance was also seen for co-trimoxazole, chloramphenicol and tetracycline [31]. A more recent ongoing multinational study (SENTRY) [32] documented a steady increase in the prevalence of penicillin resistance or intermediate level of susceptibility in *S. pneumoniae* of 16.0% and 27.8%, respectively.

The Nearchus project performed in the UK [33] showed that beta-lactamase production is the main mechanism of resistance in *H. influenzae* and *M. catarrhalis* (15% and 94%, respectively), while resistance to penicillin in *S. pneumoniae* was found in 3.4% of isolates. Another study [34] performed on a large number of *H. influenzae* and *M. catarrhalis* strains from 27 USA and 7 Canadian medical centres showed that the overall prevalence of beta-lactamase production was 33.5% in *H. influenzae* and 92.2% in *M. catarrhalis.* The authors reported > 5% resistance rate only for cefaclor (12.8%) and trimethoprim-sul-famethoxazole (16.2%) in *H. influenzae.*

A recent Italian survey, the Italian Epidemiological Observatory, monitored the resistance of the most common respiratory pathogens in a three-year systematic programme. The aims of the study were to generate national and regional data on the diffusion of resistance and to support general practitioners with epidemiological data for an empiric therapy [35]. In Italy, *S. pneumoniae* shows an overall level of intermediate resistance (reduced susceptibility) and resistance to penicillin of 12.7%, with a geographical variation ranging from 10% in the north to 17.9% in the south. Penicillin-resistant strains (MIC > 4 mg/l) were 3.8%. In this study, macrolide resistance in *S. pneumoniae* ranged from 29% to 31%, clearly exceeding the level of penicillin resistance. Penicillin-resistant strains were completely resistant to co-trimoxazole and, to a lesser extent, to erythromycin and tetracycline. In the third year of the study, 16% and 22% of *H. influenzae* and *H. parainfluenzae* strains showed beta-lactamase production, respectively, compared to 87.0% of *M. catarrhalis* (unpublished data).

Conclusions

The overall incidence of beta-lactamase-positive *Haemophilus* spp. and *M. catarrhalis,* the resistance to penicillin by means of an altered penicillin-binding protein in *S. pneumoniae,* and the increased level of macrolide resistance reduce the choice of oral antibiotics currently available for the treatment of acute respiratory tract infections, even though these maintain their usefulness against intracellular pathogens.

Cefuroxime maintains its efficacy against more than 90% of strains of *S. pneumoniae,* 97% of strains of *Haemophilus* spp. and *M. catarrhalis.* Amoxicillin had its potency restored with the addition of clavulanate, overcoming also intermediate resistance in *S. pneumoniae.* Other drugs such as cefaclor diminished, in some cases, their efficacy. Fluorquinolones (FQs) such as ciprofloxacin mantain potency against gram-negative bacteria, while the new FQs can be considered as a first-choice therapy against all resistant pathogens including *S. pneumoniae.* Finally, surveillance programmes to monitor trends of antimicrobial resistance in community-acquired respiratory tract infections (RTI) have important consequences on the empirical therapy and also bring physicians to reconsider the approach to treating RTI. Beta-lactams and macrolides are the most frequently used antibiotics in respiratory tract infections. However, beta-lactam resistance, due to both hydrolytic and non-hydrolytic mechanisms, potentially limits the apparent choice of penicillins and cephalosporins susceptible to hydrolysis. Only a few drugs maintain their efficacy because of their natural resistance to the hydrolytic mechanism of beta-lactamases (e.g. cefuroxime, ceftriaxone) or because they are protected by the addition of a beta-lactamase inhibitor (co-amoxicillin).

The frequency of resistance to macrolides in respiratory tract pathogens has limited the use of these drugs as first-choice therapy. Moreover, cross-resistant strains are isolated all around the world with increasing frequency, demonstrating that the overall key to effective treatment is the use of global and local resistance patterns to direct the choice of appropriate empirical antibiotic therapy in respiratory tract infections.

References

1. Baquero F, Alvarez ME, Canton R (1996) Bacteriologic diagnosis of respiratory tract infections. Clin Microbiol Infect 1(Suppl 2):2S10-2S15
2. Gump DW, Phillips CA, Forsyth BR, et al. (1976) Role of infection in chronic bronchitis. Am Rev Respir Dis 113:465
3. Mayaud C, Mangiapan G (1998) Role of intracellular pathogens in respiratory tract infections. Clin Microbiol Infect 4(Suppl 4):4S14-4S22
4. Blasi F, Legnani D, Lombardo V, et al. (1993) *Chlamydia pneumoniae* infection in acute exacerbations of COPD. Eur Respir J 6:19-22
5. Tager D, Speizer TE (1975) The role of infection in chronic bronchitis. N Engl J Med 292:563-571
6. Krasemann C, Koch RC (1991) Microrganismi patogeni nella bronchite cronica. In: Ciprofloxacin in pulmonology symposium, Lausanne, June 1990. Edizioni Minerva Medica, pp 3-6
7. Pellegrino MB, Privitera A, Primavera A, Puntorieri M, Nicoletti A, Stefani S, Nicoletti G (1992) Microbiological considerations of the etiological agents of lower respiratory tract infections. J Chemother 4(4):211-215
8. Grossman RF (1999) Management of acute exacerbation of chronic bronchitis. Can Respir J 6(Suppl A):40A-50A
9. Smith CB, Golden CA, Kanner RE, Renzetti AD (1976) *Haemophilus influenzae* and *Haemophilus parainfluenzae* in chronic obstructive pulmonary diseases. Lancet 1:1253-1255
10. Rhind GB, Gould GA, Ahmad F, Croughan MJ, Calder MA (1985) *Haemophilus influenzae* and *H. parainfluenzae* respiratory infections: comparison of clinical features. BMJ 291:707-708
11. Devalia JL, Grady D, Harmanyeri Y, Tabaqchali S, Davies RJ (1989) Histamine synthesis by respiratory tract micro-organisms: possible role in pathogenicity. J Clin Pathol 42:516-522
12. Cole P (1989) Host-microbe relationship in chronic respiratory infections. Respiration 55(Suppl 1):5-8
13. Stefani S, Russo G, Schito GC, Varaldo PE, Filadoro F, Satta G, Covelli I, Varanese L (1993) Multicenter study of isolation and resistance to some antibiotics of *Branhamella catarrhalis* In: Recent Advances in Chemotherapy, Proceedings of 18th ICC, Stockholm 1993. American Society for Microbiology, Washington DC, pp 308-309
14. McGregor K, Chang BJ, Mee BJ, Riley TV (1998) *Moraxella catarrhalis*: clinical significance, antimicrobial susceptibility and BRO beta-lactamases. Eur J Clin Microbiol Infect Dis 17: 219-234
15. Anon R (1982) *Branhamella catarrhalis*: pathogen or opportunistic? Lancet 1:1056
16. Catlin BW (1990) *Branhamella catarrhalis*: an organism gaining respect as a pathogen. Clin Microbiol Rev 3:292-320

17. Stefani S, Pellegrino MB, Russo G, Nicoletti G (1991) Direct and indirect pathogenicity of beta-lactamase producing bacteria in respiratory tract infections in children. Drugs 42(Suppl 4):14-18

18. Eller J, Aja Ede MD, Schaberg T, Niederman MS, Mauch H, Lode H (1998) Infective exacerbations of chronic bronchitis. Chest 113:1542-1548

19. Miravitlles M, Espinosa C, Fernandez-Laso E, Martos JA, Maldonado JA, Gallego M (1999) Relationship between bacterial flora in sputum and functional impairment in patients with acute exacerbations of COPD. Study Group of Bacterial Infection in COPD. Chest 116(1):40-46

20. Cosentini R, Tarsia P, Blasi F (1999) *Chlamydia pneumoniae:* clinical characteristics of acute respiratory infections. In: Allegra L, Blasi F (eds) *Chlamydia pneumoniae* – The lung and the heart. Springer, Berlin Heidelberg New York, pp 70-79

21. Forsgren JA, Samuelson A, Ahlin A, Jonasson J, Rynnel-Dagoo B, Lindberg A (1994) *Haemophilus influenzae* resides and multiplies intracellularly in human adenoid tissue as demonstrated by in situ hybridization and bacterial viability assay. Infect Immun 62:673-679

22. Bresser P, van Alphen L, Habets FJ, Hart AA, Dankert J, Jansen M, Lutter R (1997) Persisting *Haemophilus influenzae* strains induce lower levels of interleukin-6 and interleukin-8 in H292 lung epithelial cells than non-persisting strains. Eur Respir J 10:2319-2326

23. Brunham RC, Plummer FA, Stephens RS (1993) Bacterial antigenic variation, host immune response, and pathogen-host coevolution. Infect Immun 61:2273- 2276

24. Groenenveld K, van Alphen C, Voorter C, Eijk PP, Jansen HM, Zanen HC (1989) Antigenic drift of *Haemophilus influenzae* in patients with chronic obstructive pulmonary disease. Infect Immun 57:3038-3044

25. Groeneveld K, van Alphen L, Eijk PP, Visschers G, Jansen HM, Zanen HC (1990) Endogenous and exogenous reinfections by *Haemophilus influenzae* in patients with chronic obstructive pulmonary disease: the effect of antibiotic treatment on persistence. J Infect Dis 161:512-517

26. Hood DW, Deadman ME, Jennings MP, Bisercic M, Fleischmann RD, Venter JC, Moxon ER (1996) DNA repeats identify novel virulence genes in *Haemophilus influenzae.* Proc Natl Acad Sci USA 93:1121-1125

27. van Belkum A, Scherer S, Van Leeuwen W, Willemse D, van Alpèhen L, Verbrugh H (1997) Variable number of tandem repeats in clinical strains of *Haemophilus influenzae.* Infect Immun 65:5017-5027

28. Gump DW, Christmas WA, Forsyth BR, Phillips CA, Stouch WH (1973) Serum and secretory antibodies in patient with chronic bronchitis. Arch Intern Med 132:847-851

29. Privitera A, Licciardello L, Giannino V, Agodi A, Rappazzo G, Nicoletti G, Stefani S (1998) Molecular epidemiology and phylogenetic analysis of *Haemophilus parainfluenzae* from chronic obstructive pulmonary diseases exacerbations. Eur J Epidemiol 14:405-412

30. Gruneberg RN, Felmingham D and the Alexander Project Group (1996) Results of the Alexander Project: a continuing, multicenter study of the antimicrobial susceptibility of community-acquired lower respiratory tract bacterial pathogens. Diagn Microbiol Infect Dis 25:169-181

31. Garau J (1999) Basic empiric treatment choices for respiratory tract infection on the results of the Alexander Project. J Chemotherapy 11(1):51-55

32. Doern GV, Pfaller MA, Kugler K, Freeman J, Jones RN (1998) Prevalence of antimicrobial resistance among respiratory tract isolates of *Streptococcus pneumoniae* in North America: 1997 results from the SENTRY antimicrobial surveillance program. Clin Infect Dis 27:764-770

33. Gruneberg RN, Felmingham D, Harding I, Shrimpton SB, Nathwani A (1998) The Nearchus project: antibiotic susceptibility of respiratory pathogens and clinical outcome in lower respiratory tract infections at 27 centres in the UK. Int J Antimicrob Agents 10:127-133

34. Doern GV, Jones RN, Pfaller MA, Kugler K, and The Sentry Participants Group (1997) *Haemophilus influenzae* and *Moraxella catarrhalis* from patients with community-acquired respiratory tract infections: antimicrobial susceptibility patterns from the SENTRY antimicrobial surveillance program (United States and Canada 1997). Antimicrob Agents Chemother 43:385-389

35. Schito GC, Nicoletti G (1998) Osservatorio Epidemiologico Italiano per il rilevamento delle resistenze ai farmaci antimicrobici nei patogeni batterici delle vie respiratorie. Gior Ital Microbiol Med Odont Clin II(2):5-43

Severe Acute Exacerbations of COPD: Epidemiology and Antimicrobial Treatment

S. Ewig[1], N. Soler[2], A. Torres[2]

Introduction

Severity criteria for exacerbations of chronic obstructive pulmonary disease (COPD) have not yet been defined as they have for pneumonia. Therefore, investigators have usually adopted pragmatic criteria to define their study populations according to the subject of the study. For example, studies addressing modalities of ventilatory support have used acute severe hypoxemia and/or hypercapnic failure as entry criteria [1-5]. Most studies evaluating antimicrobial treatment have characterized the populations studied by the severity of airflow limitation in stable states and/or during exacerbations [6-9]. However, patients with severe airflow limitation (e.g. forced expiratory volume in one second – FEV_1 – < 35% predicted) in stable states or during an exacerbation may or may not present with acute respiratory failure and vice versa. On the other hand, a recent study has provided evidence that patients with severe airflow limitation may be more likely to have an infection by gram-negative enterobacteriaceae (GNEB) or *Pseudomonas aeruginosa* [9] but it is not known whether the type of pathogen independently predicts severe exacerbations.

Thus, at present it seems reasonable to confine the term "severe COPD exacerbation" to patients requiring admission to an intensive care unit (ICU) according to clinical judgment. In order to establish a more objective definition of severe exacerbations, it will be crucial in future trials to properly define patients requiring ICU admission. In the meantime, the following criteria advanced by the American Thoracic Society (ATS) [10] may be useful:
1. Severe dsypnea that responds inadequately to initial emergency therapy;
2. Confusion, lethargy, or respiratory muscle fatigue;
3. Persistent or worsening hypoxemia, despite supplemental oxygen or severe/worsening respiratory acidosis (pH < 7.30); and
4. Requirement of assisted mechanical ventilation (invasive or noninvasive techniques).

---

[1] Department of Internal Medicine and Respiratory Diseases, University of Bonn, Sigmund Freud Strasse 25, 53105 Bonn, Germany; [2] Hospital Clinic i Provincial, Department of Respiratory Diseases and Allergology, University of Barcelona, Barcelona, Spain

Epidemiology

Incidence

The incidence of severe acute COPD exacerbations requiring ICU admission is not known. However, it is probable that a considerable part of patients with advanced COPD will require ICU treatment at any time during the course of the disease.

Prognosis

In-hospital mortality of acute COPD exacerbations requiring hospitalization ranged between 11% and 14% [11,12]. Mortality associated with acute hypercapnic failure (mostly treated without assisted ventilation) was 12% [1]. Patients requiring intubation and mechanical ventilation tended to have a higher mortality than those without assisted ventilation (14%-32%) [3-5]. This was apparently not true for patients requiring noninvasive ventilation (NIPPV), with associated mortality rates ranging between 6% and 12% [1, 4].

The long-term prognosis after hospital discharge is considerably worse. In the largest recent study of 1016 patients hospitalized with severe hypercapnic exacerbations, in-hospital mortality rate was 11% but 2-year mortality was 49%. In addition, survivors were at high risk of requiring care in a nursing home or readmission to the hospital within the next six months [12].

The independent impact of infections on mortality has only rarely been assessed. In patients with severe acute exacerbations and hypercapnic failure ($pCO_2 \geq 50$ mm Hg) requiring hospitalization, prognostic factors predicting in-hospital outcome were severity of illness, body mass index, age, prior functional status, PaO_2/F_IO_2, serum albumin, and the presence of cor pulmonale. Infection as a cause of an acute episode of COPD was not predictive [12]. In two studies assessing the microbiology of severe COPD exacerbations requiring mechanical ventilation, mortality was low (11% and 6%) [13, 14]. These data cast doubt that infection by itself increases the risk of death. Nevertheless, the independent role of specific pathogens has not been specifically addressed in terms of prognosis.

Microbiology

The microbiology of severe acute COPD exacerbations requiring mechanical ventilation has been assessed in only two studies [13, 14], including a recent study conducted at the Hospital Clinic in Barcelona, Spain [14]. Both studies used quantitative cultures. These studies confirmed the following observations:
1. Around 50% of patients have potentially pathogenic microorganisms (PPMs) in respiratory secretions;
2. More than half of these patients have PPMs in amounts equal to or higher than that known to be present in pneumonia;
3. Non-PPMs are also present in significant amounts.

The studies differed mainly in the proportion of potentially drug-resistant isolates. Whereas these were present only exceptionally in the study by Fagon, et al. [13], we found these pathogens to be thrice as common (22% versus 7% of pathogens) [14]. Our study offered two additional insights:

1. Only 12% of patients had no evidence of infection in lower respiratory tract samples despite absence of any antimicrobial pretreatment; with the additional use of serology the proportion of patients with a probable infectious cause of exacerbation increased from 52% to 72%;

2. *Chlamydia pneumonia* accounted for the majority of "atypical" bacterial pathogens, whereas influenza virus was the most common viral isolate.

From these studies, it is difficult to judge whether microbial patterns of severe exacerbations differ from those of less severe episodes. In both nonsevere and severe exacerbations, endogenous community pathogens seem to predominate. However, this view has recently been challenged by a study demonstrating that GNEB and *Pseudomonas aeruginosa* accounted for two-thirds of pathogens in hospitalized patients with severe airflow limitations in the stable state ($FEV_1 < 35\%$ predicted) [9], whereas endogenous community pathogens were preponderant in mild COPD ($FEV_1 \geq \%$ predicted).

In our study, there was no significant association between microbial patterns and FEV_1, nevertheless, we also found a high incidence of potentially drug-resistant microorganisms [14]. The proportion of *Chlamydia pneumoniae* was higher than that in previous studies in ambulatory and hospitalized patients with acute exacerbations (18% of patients versus 4%-5%) [15, 16], but this finding remains to be confirmed in further studies. The proportion of viral infections was not different from that in nonsevere courses [17]. Clearly, further studies are required to clarify the relative frequencies of different pathogens in nonsevere and severe exacerbations.

Management

Indications for Antimicrobial Treatment

Antimicrobial treatment for acute exacerbations of COPD remains a controversial subject. In fact, evidence for its effectiveness in this setting is scarce. A recent metanalysis of nine placebo-controlled studies published between 1957 and 1992 showed a small but statistically significant improvement due to antimicrobial treatment [18]. However, the largest study which provided the most conclusive evidence in favor of antibiotics, at least in the subgroup presenting with increased dyspnea, sputum volume and sputum purulence (the so-called Anthonisen-type-I exacerbation), included mainly patients with moderate to severe airflow limitation at baseline (predicted mean FEV_1 34% ± 14%) [7]. In contrast, the most recent placebo-controlled study including mild to moderate COPD patients did not find any benefit for antimicrobial treatment [8]. These studies suggest that bronchial mucosal infection may be self-limiting in most instances, especially in mild-to-moderately ill patients but may require antimicrobial treatment in the more severely ill.

On the other hand, provocative data were presented by Fagon, et al. in patients with severe exacerbations requiring mechanical ventilation [13]. In this study, mortality rates, duration of mechanical ventilation, and duration of hospitalization were not significantly different between patients with positive microbiology as assessed by the protected specimen brush (PSB) and patients without any bacterial pathogen. Moreover, in the latter patients, outcome parameters were similar whether or not antimicrobial treatment was administered. In view of these results, the authors questioned the predominant role of bacterial infection in the pathogenesis and course of acute exacerbations. However, these data must be interpreted with great caution since the populations studied were small and antimicrobial treatment was not randomized. In fact, there was at least a trend for a longer duration of mechanical ventilation and hospitalization of approximately 2-3 days in patients with evidence for an infectious bacterial etiology. Moreover, as stated previously, this study had a very low incidence of potentially drug-resistant microorganisms and may, therefore, not be comparable to other populations.

We recently carried out a study to assess the effect of antimicrobial treatment in terms of bacterial load reduction and bacterial eradication [19]. The population studied was that described in Table 1; the effect of antimicrobial treatment was assessed regardless of colony counts. Resistance was common among the pathogens isolated. All five isolates of *Streptococcus pneumoniae* were resistant to penicillin, 4 of 12 isolates of *Haemophilus influenzae* and 4 of 5 of *Moraxella catarrhalis* produced beta-lactamases, and 4 of 9 isolates of *Pseudomonas* spp. as well as 1 of 2 of *Stenotrophomonas maltophilia* were multiresistant. Overall, in those patients receiving a repeated examination after 72 h, the bacterial load could be significantly reduced but 23% of pathogens persisted. Bacterial persistance was significantly associated with inappropriate initial antimicrobial treatment. However, it was not possible to demonstrate a significantly worse outcome in patients with bacterial persistance after 72 h in terms of duration of mechanical ventilation, ICU stay, and mortality. However, two patients with persistant, potentially drug-resistant microorganisms developed pneumonia, and of these, one died. These results demonstrate that (1) appropriate antimicrobial treatment is effective in eradicating bacterial pathogens, (2) bacterial persistance is a consequence of inappropriate antimicrobial treatment, and (3) bacterial persistance may bear significant hazards. Whether a significant reduction of bacterial load is equally effective as eradication in terms of outcome remains to be studied.

Since current evidence supports antimicrobial treatment in subgroups of patients, especially the more severely ill, and in view of the severity of the present complication as well as the underlying condition, we advocate initial empiric antimicrobial treatment in all patients with severe acute COPD exacerbations. In patients without prior ambulatory antimicrobial treatment, negative cultures of lower respiratory tract secretions, and lack of indirect evidence for bacterial infection (such as purulent sputum, leucocytosis, or elevated C-reactive protein) antimicrobial treatment may be stopped. However, since atypical bacterial pathogens may be present in these patients, coverage of these pathogens may be considered.

Table 1. Comparison of microbial patterns in acute COPD exacerbations requiring mechanical ventilation, according to two studies. Fagon, et al. [13] reported only microorganisms 10^2 cfu/ml. Soler, et al. [14] reported microorganisms above predefined cut-offs: PSB (protected specimen brush) $\geq 10^2$ cfu/ml; BAL (bronchoalveolar lavage) $\geq 10^3$ cfu/ml; and tracheobronchial aspirates $\geq 10^5$ cfu/ml

Microorganism	Fagon, et al. [13] (n = 54)[a]	Soler, et al. [14] (n = 50)[b]
PPMs: endogenous community pathogens		
Haemophilus influenzae	6	11
Streptococcus pneumoniae	7	4
Moraxella catarrhalis	3	4
Staphylococcus aureus	4	-
PPMs: GNEB	5	4
PPMs: potentially drug-resistant microorganisms		
Pseudomonas spp.	3*	9*
Stenotrophomonas maltophilia	-*	2*
Non-PPMs		
Other streptococci	4	NR
Corynebacterium spp.	1	NR
Haemophilus parainfluenzae	11	NR
Other bacteria		
Chlamydia pneumoniae	NI	7
Chlamydia psittaci	NI	1
Coxiella burnetii	NI	1
Respiratory viruses		
Influenza virus	NI	5
Respiratory syncitial virus	NI	1

PPMs, potentially pathogenic microorganisms; *GNEB*, gram-negative enterobacteriaceae; *NI*, not investigated; *NR*, not reported; * significantly different at $p < 0.05$; [a]27 patients with 44 pathogens; [b]36 patients with 49 pathogens

Diagnostic Evaluation

Current evidence clearly supports the importance of obtaining valid lower respiratory tract samples for culture in order to establish the presence of bacterial pathogens and their susceptibility patterns. For example, in our study, results of diagnostic evaluation directed a change in antimicrobial treatment in 36% of cases [19].

Although sputum is an impure sample, sputum analysis may be the only diagnostic technique applicable in nonintubated patients with severe dyspnea. The easiest way to obtain a lower respiratory tract sample in intubated patients is to retrieve a tracheobronchial aspirate (TBAS). The bronchoscopically retrieved protected specimen brush (PSB) is probably more specific but less sensitive. Bronchoalveolar lavage (BAL) samples a large area of the lung (around 1%) but is more representative for lung parenchyma rather than tracheobronchial mucosa. Tracheobronchial aspiration has the great advantage of being repeatable and may be used to assess the effect of antimicrobial treatment after 72 h. The demonstration of a positive IgM for *Mycoplasma pneumoniae* or *Chlamydia pneumoniae* may be occasionally useful. However, since paired samples are required in most instances to obtain vaild results, serology is not often helpful in individual cases. The value of virus cultures from nasopharyngeal swabs or washings or from bronchoalveolar lavage fluid (BALF) has not been systematically elucidated. However, in our experience, bacterial overgrowth precludes valid results in a considerable number of instances.

Choice of Initial Antimicrobial Treatment Regimen

Empiric initial antimicrobial treatment should be designed according to general microbial and susceptibility patterns reported in the literature as well as – ideally – to those observed in the actual treatment center. For example, the antimicrobial regimen should cover endogenous community pathogens such as *Streptococcus pneumoniae, Haemophilus influenzae, Staphylococcus aureus*, and *Moraxella catarrhalis* as well as gram-negative enteric enterobacteriaceae (GNEB). Evidently, this can only be accomplished taking into account the local incidence of *Streptococcus pneumoniae* resistant to penicillin and macrolides, of ß-lactamase-producing strains of *Haemophilus influenzae* and *Moraxella catarrhalis*, and of extended spectrum β-lactamase-producing strains (ESBL) of GNEB.

In regions with a low prevalence of penicillin-resistant pneumococci, aminopenicillin plus β-lactamase inhibitor may still be an appropriate choice. Using this regimen, β-lactamase-producing *Haemophilus influenzae* and *Moraxella catarrhalis* would also be covered. Otherwise, a third-generation cephalosporin or a new quinolone such as levofloxacin may be the preferred regimen. Quinolones offer the additional advantage of covering atypical bacterial pathogens. This may also be afforded by a combination of a third-generation cephalosporin and a newer macrolide (clarithromycin, roxithromycin, azithromycin).

Whereas regular coverage of potentially drug-resistant microorganisms is probably not necessary, we advocate administering an antipseudomonal regimen to any patient previously known to be colonized with *Pseudomonas aeruginosa*. This recommendation is based on the notion that sterilization of the airways in a patient colonized by this pathogen is unlikely to occur more than transiently as a result of previous antimicrobial treatment. Therefore, the occurence of this pathogen in a corresponding patient with an acute exacerbation would be highly probable. Effective antipseudomonal treatment will require combination regimen including antipseudomonal third-generation cephalosporin (ceftazidime) or acylureidopenicillin (piperacillin ± β-lactamase inhibitor), plus aminoglycoside (tobramycin or amikacin) or plus ciprofloxacin.

Severe acute exacerbations usually require an intravenous administration of antimicrobial agents. However, antimicrobial treatment should be switched to oral formulations as soon as possible. The duration of antimicrobial treatment is not standardized, and data to support a distinct recommendation are not available. In our experience, microorganisms susceptible to the administered drugs can be eradicated within 72 h [19]. However, in view of possible relapses and potentially drug-resistant microorganisms, it seems reasonable to administer antimicrobial treatment for 7-10 days.

Appropriate antimicrobial agents and combination regimen for severe acute COPD exacerbations are summarized in Table 2.

Table 2. Antimicrobial agents for the treatment of acute severe COPD exacerbations

Antimicrobial agent	Dosage	Comments
Aminopenicillin/ß-lactamase inhibitor		
Amoxicillin/clavulanic acid	3 x 2.2 g	
Acylureidopenicillins		
Piperacillin/tazobactam	3-4 x 4 g / 0.5 g	
Third-generation cephalosporins		Active against drug-resistant pneumococci
Cefotaxime	3 x 2 g	
Ceftriaxone	1-2 x 1 g	
Ceftazidime	3 x 2 g	Antipseudomonal cephalosporin
Fourth-generation cephalosporins		
Cefepime	2 x 2 g	Antipseudomonal cephalosporin
Carbapenems		
Imipenem/cilastatin	3-4 x 1 g	
Meropenem	3-4 x 1 g	
Macrolides		Active against atypical bacterial pathogens
Erythromycin	3-4 x 1 g	Poor activity against *Haemophilus influenzae*
Azithromycin	1 x 500 mg day 1, 1 x 250 mg days 2-5	Only oral formulation; increased activity against *Haemophilus influenzae*
Aminoglycosides		Poor penetration in lung tissue and respiratory secretions
Tobramycin	1 x 5-7 mg/kg	
Amikacin	1 x 15 mg/kg	
Quinolones		Excellent penetration in lung tissues and respiratory secretions; active against atypical bacterial pathogens
Ciprofloxacin	3 x 400 mg	Best antipseudomonal activity within quinolone group
Levofloxacin	1 x 500 mg	Increased activity against gram-positive pathogens

Conclusions

The present review indicates that virtually all important issues in the epidemiology and management of severe acute COPD exacerbations remain unsettled. Perhaps the most important area of future research is to appropriately define COPD exacerbations in general and severity criteria of this condition in particular, so that future trials evaluating microbial and susceptibility patterns as well as antimicrobial treatment may be comparable.

While awaiting the results of these studies, in our view, diagnostic evaluation at least by tracheobronchial aspiration and immediate empiric antimicrobial treatment remain the mainstay for a favorable outcome in patients with acute exacerbations requiring ICU admission. General and local microbial and susceptibility patterns should form the basis for designing these empiric regimens and should be specifically modified according to the diagnostic results.

References

1. Jeffrey AA, Warren PW, Flenley DC (1992) Acute hypercapnic respiratory failure in patients with chronic obstructive lung disease: risk factors and use of guidelines for management. Thorax 47:34-40
2. Bott J, Carroll MP, Conway JH, Keilty SE, Ward EM, Brown AM, Paul EA, Elliott MW, Godfrey RC, Wedzicha JA (1993) Randomized controlled trial of nasal ventilation in acute ventilatory failure due to chronic obstructive airways disease. Lancet 341:1555-1557
3. Seneff MG, Wagner DP, Wagner RP, et al. (1995) Hospital and 1-year survival of patients admitted to intensive care units with acute exacerbations of chronic obstructive pulmonary disease. JAMA 274:1852-1857
4. Brochard L, Mancebo J, Wysocki M, et al. (1995) Noninasive ventilation for acute exacerbations of chronic obstructive pulmonary disease. N Engl J Med 333:817-822
5. Moran JL, Green JV, Homan SD, Lesson RJ, Leppard PI (1998) Acute exacerbations of chronic obstructive pulmonary disease and mechanical ventilation: a reevaluation. Crit Care Med 26:71-78
6. Nicotra MB, Rivera M, Awe RJ (1982) Antibiotic therapy of acute exacerbations of chronic bronchitis. Ann Intern Med 97:18-21
7. Anthonisen NR, Manfreda J, Warren CPW, Hershfield ES, Harding GKM, Nelson NA (1987) Antibiotic therapy in exacerbations of chronic obstructive pulmonary disease. Ann Intern Med 106:196-204
8. Sachs APE, Koeter GH, Groenier KH, van der Waaij D, Schiphuis J, Meyboom-de Jong B (1995) Changes in symptoms, peak expiratory flow, and sputum flora during treatment with antibiotics of exacerbations in patients with chronic obstructive pulmonary disease in general practice. Thorax 50:758-763
9. Eller J, Ede A, Schaberg T, Niederman MS, Mauch H, Lode H (1998) Infective exacerbations of chronic bronchitis. Relation between bacteriology etiology and lung function. Chest 113:1542-1548
10. American Thoracic Society Statement (1995) Standards for the diagnosis and care of patients with chronic obstructive pulmonary disease. Am J Respir Crit Care Med 152:S97-S106

11. Fuso L, Incalzi RA, Pistelli R, Muzzolon R, Valente S, Pagliari G, Gliozzi F, Ciappi G (1995) Predicting mortality of patients hospitalized for acutely exacerbated chronic obstructive pulmonary disease. Am J Med 98:272-277

12. Connors AF, Dawson NV, Thomas C, Harrell FE Jr, Desbiens N, Fulkerson WJ, Kussin P, Bellamy P, Goldman L, Knaus WA for the SUPPORT Investigators (1996) Outcomes following acute exacerbation of severe chronic obstructive lung disease. Am J Respir Crit Care Med 154:959-967

13. Fagon JY, Chastre J, Trouillet JL, Domart Y, Dombret MC, Bornet M, Gibert C (1990) Characterization of distal bronchial microflora during acute exacerbations of chronic bronchitis. Am Rev Respir Dis 142:1004-1008

14. Soler N, Torres A, Ewig S, Gonzalez J, Celis R, El-Ebiary M, Hernandez C, Rodriguez-Roisin R (1998) Bronchial microbial patterns in severe exacerbations of chronic obstructive pulmonary disease (COPD) requiring mechanical ventilation. Am J Respir Crit Care Med 157:1498-1505

15. Beaty CD, Grayston JT, Wang SP, Kuo CC, Reto CS, Martin TR (1991) *Chlamydia pneumoniae*, strain TWAR, infection in patients with chronic obstructive pulmonary disease. Am Rev Respir Dis 144:1408-1410

16. Blasi F, Legnani D, Lombardo VM, Negretto GG, Magliano E, Pozzoli, Chiodo F, Fasoli F, Allegra L (1993) *Chlamydia pneumoniae* infection in acute exacerbations of COPD. Eur Respir J 6:19-22

17. Gump DW, Phillips CA, Forsyth BR, McIntosh K, Lamborn KR, Stouch WH (1976) Role of infection in chronic bronchitis. Am Rev Respir Dis 113:465-474

18. Saint S, Bent S, Vittinghoff E, Grady D (1995) Antibiotics in chronic obstructive pulmonary disease exacerbations. A meta-analysis. JAMA 273:957-960

19. Ewig S, Soler N, Gonzalez J, El-Ebiary M, Celis R, Torres A (2000) Evaluation of antimicrobial treatment in mechanically ventilated patients with severe COPD exacerbations. Crit Care Med (*in press*)

Antibiotics in the Treatment of Acute Exacerbations of Chronic Bronchitis: A Review of Controlled Clinical Trials

F. BLASI[1], R. COSENTINI[2]

Introduction

The term chronic bronchitis is clinically defined as the presence of excess mucus secretion, causing productive cough on most days for at least three months of the year for at least 2 consecutive years and when other causes of cough have been excluded [1]. When airway obstruction is also present, the term chronic obstructive pulmonary disease (COPD) is applied. The true epidemiological impact of COPD is unknown, but it is estimated that in the United States approximately 1 of 5 adult subjects are affected, and that this disease is the fourth leading cause of mortality [2, 3].

During the natural course of the disease, all patients with chronic bronchitis experience acute exacerbations. The diagnosis of an acute exacerbation rests on clinical criteria such as history of increased cough, increased sputum volume and purulence, and worsening dyspnoea [4]. The causes triggering an acute exacerbation are generally multifactorial and commonly include a combination of smoking habits, environmental irritants and infection [5]. It is thought that up to 70% of infectious cases are caused by bacteria, the remainder being attributable to "atypical" pathogens such as viruses, *Mycoplasma pneumoniae*, and *Chlamydia pneumoniae* [6]. However, the role of bacterial infections in acute exacerbations of chronic bronchitis is still controversial. In this setting, findings commonly associated with infection, such as fever and leukocytosis, are often absent. Notwithstanding the use of bacterial culture techniques and increased antibody titres as markers of acute infection, an association between exacerbations and acute bacterial infection has not been clearly demonstrated [5, 7, 8]. Nevertheless, a correlation between repeated infections and a more rapid decline in respiratory function has been shown, and acute infections may initiate a vicious circle leading to a pattern of repetitive infective exacerbations [9, 10].

Among bacterial agents, *Haemophilus influenzae*, *Streptococcus pneumoniae*, and *Moraxella catarrhalis* are consistently reported as the three most common

---

[1] Institute of Respiratory Diseases, University of Milan, IRCCS Ospedale Maggiore, Milan, Italy; [2] Division of Emergency Medicine, IRCCS Ospedale Maggiore, Milan, Italy

pathogens causing acute exacerbations of chronic bronchitis [4, 6, 11]. *Haemophilus influenzae* is the most common pathogen isolated from expectorated sputum and is held to be responsible for 35%-50% of exacerbations, whereas recent clinical trials confirm that *Streptococcus pneumoniae* is responsible for 20% or less of exacerbations [6, 12, 13]. Viruses and *Mycoplasma pneumoniae* account for approximately one-third of acute exacerbations [6] and in roughly 5% of patients with chronic bronchitis exacerbations are caused by *Chlamydia pneumoniae* infection [14].

Antibiotics and AECB

If the role of bacterial infections is still controversial, the efficacy of antimicrobial therapy in acute exacerbations of chronic bronchitis (AECB) is even more *uncertain*. Two approaches have been used in order to evaluate the effect of antibiotics on the natural history of AECB and chronic bronchitis. The first is the prophylactic use of antibiotics that should lead to a decrease in number and frequency of AECB. Many studies tried to address this issue; among these, nine were placebo-controlled studies involving more than 25 patients (Table 1) [15-23].

Murphy and Sethi [24] further analysed those trials showing a benefit from antibiotic prophylaxis. They observed that patients who were most likely to expe-

Table 1. Placebo-controlled clinical trials of chemoprophylaxis for acute exacerbations of chronic bronchitis

Trial	Benefit
The Working Party on Trials of Chemotherapy in Early Chronic Bronchitis of The Medical Research Council [15]	No reduction in the frequency of exacerbations; Less time lost from work in the antibiotic group
Davis, et al. [16]	No reduction in the frequency of exacerbations
Priedie, et al. [17]	No reduction in the frequency of exacerbations
Francis, Spicer [18]	No reduction in the frequency of exacerbations; less time lost from work in the antibiotic group
Johnston, et al. [19]	No reduction in the frequency of exacerbations;
Davis, et al. [20]	Statistically significant reduction in the frequency of exacerbations
Buchanan, et al. [21]	Statistically significant reduction in the frequency of exacerbations
Pines [22]	Statistically significant reduction in the frequency of exacerbations
Johnston, et al. [23]	Statistically significant reduction in the frequency of exacerbations

rience beneficial effects of prophylaxis were those with a more relevant clinical impairment (as determined by number of past exacerbations). Patients who experienced many exacerbations (approximately four or more per year) were most likely to benefit from antibiotic prophylaxis whereas this effect was less likely to occur in patients with one or two exacerbations per year. In summary, the available studies indicate that antibiotic prophylaxis strategy should be limited to patients with a more severe clinical impairment as determined by number of exacerbation in the previous years.

The other possible approach in evaluating the role of antibiotic treatment in exacerbations of chronic bronchitis is to assess the efficacy of antibiotic therapy on the severity and course of a single exacerbation, after its onset. At least ten placebo-controlled studies have been performed to evaluate the possible beneficial effects of antibiotic treatment in patients with acute exacerbations of chronic bronchitis [25-34].

A recent meta-analysis of nine randomised, placebo-controlled trials [25-32, 34] of patients on antibiotic treatment in AECB demonstrated only a small but statistically significant improvement attributable to antimicrobial therapy [35]. Table 2 summarises the results of these placebo-controlled studies. Major difficulties in defining the true value of antibiotic treatment are the lack of unifying definitions of an exacerbation as well as the heterogeneity of chronic bronchitis patients in terms of severity of the underlying disease. Moreover, in most of the placebo-controlled studies tetracyclines and co-trimoxazole were used. These drugs are probably less active than newer antibiotics that possess a wider bacterial spectrum and/or better pharmacokinetics. It is also important to bear in mind that both baseline severity and exacerbation severity may be associated with unusual bacterial aetiologies such as *Pseudomonas aeruginosa* [36]. Antibiotic-associated improvement may be therefore particularly significant in patients with greater baseline pulmonary dysfunction although it is still unclear whether all COPD patients need antibiotic treatment.

The recommendations of the European Respiratory Society [37] move along these lines: the need to assess exacerbation severity and functional impairment is beginning to be appreciated. Antibiotic therapy is always recommended in severe exacerbations, but also in non-severe exacerbations if increases in sputum purulence and volume are present together with worsening dyspnoea. Treatment should always last at least 7 days.

The choice of the antibiotic employed depends on the habitual prescribing behaviour of the clinician and, when available, local pathogen epidemiological considerations, as well as information on previous antibiotic failures. The impact on the cost of treatment differs widely according to the antibiotic employed, although drug expenses never account for more than 10%-16% of total costs. The rate of relapse following antibiotic treatment is a fundamental determinant of expenses, because patients with more relapses consume more health resources. On the other hand, slow remission of an exacerbation also expands total treatment expenses.

Comparing the time span between exacerbations, after the use of so-called first choice (amoxicillin, tetracycline, erythromycin, or co-trimoxazole), second

Table 2. Placebo-controlled clinical trials of antibiotic treatment in acute exacerbations of chronic bronchitis

Reference	Patients (n)	Exacerbations (n)	Treatment	Outcome measures	Results
Elmes, et al. [25]	88	113	Oxytetracycline	Days of illness	The treated group lost on the average 5.2 fewer days from work per exacerbation compared with the placebo group
Berry, et al. [26]	53	53	Oxytetracycline	Severity score	Treated patients recovered sooner and deteriorated less often than the controls. This advantage was statistically significant for patients with moderately severe attacks but not for those with mild attacks
Fear, Edwards [27]	62	119	Oxytetracycline	Duration of exacerbation, clinical response	The duration of the relapses in the treated patients was reduced by half
Elmes, et al. [28]	56	56	Ampicillin	Mortality, length of hospital stay, relapses in hospital, relapses after discharge, change in PEFR	No conclusive evidence that ampicillin was beneficial. Higher (not significantly) mortality in the control group. In-hospital relapses occurred significantly more often in the control group. Higher (not significantly) increase in PEFR in the treated group
Petersen, et al. [29]	19	19	Chloramphenicol	Change in lung function tests	The lung function tests showed no significantly different response to treatment
Pines, et al. [30]	259	259	Tetracycline (89) or chloramphenicol (84)	Clinical score, change in PEFR	Clinically, antibiotic treatment was superior to placebo. Patients treated with chloramphenicol benefited little more than those given tetracycline, except that chloramphenicol was much better tolerated. PEFR improved by a mean 10.7%, 12.6%, and 4.7% in tetracycline, chloramphenicol and placebo groups, respectively
Nicotra, et al. [31]	40	40	Tetracycline	PaO_2, change in PEFR	More pronounced improvement in oxygenation occurred in the tetracycline group. No difference in PEFR changes
Anthonisen, et al. [32]	173	362	Trimethoprim-sulfamethoxazole, amoxicillin or doxycycline	Clinical response, change in lung function tests	The success rate with placebo was 55% and with antibiotic 68%. The rate of failure with deterioration was 19% with placebo and 10% with antibiotic. There was a significant benefit associated with antibiotic. PEFR recovered more rapidly with antibiotic treatment than with placebo. Type 1 exacerbations (increased dyspnoea, sputum volume, and sputum purulence) showed a relatively large advantage for antibiotic therapy
Allegra, et al. [33]	335	335	Amoxicillin/clavulanic acid (7:1)	Clinical score, change in lung function tests	The failure rate with placebo was 49.7% and with antibiotic 13.6%. FEV₁ recovered more rapidly with antibiotic than with placebo
Jorgensen, et al. [34]	268	268	Amoxicillin	Clinical response, change in PEFR	No difference in terms of success rate and PEFR increase

PEFR, peak expiratory flow rate; FEV_1, forced expiratory volume in one second choice (oral cephalosporins), or third choice antibiotics (co-amoxiclav, ciprofloxacin and azithromycin), it has been shown that first and second line drugs allow exacerbation-free intervals of 18.3 and 23.7 weeks, respectively, whereas third choice antibiotics gave an interval of 33 weeks [38].

A New Insight in an Old Study

In order to provide additional proof of the utility of antibiotic treatment in AECB, we retrospectively extended the analysis of a previously reported study carried out on a population of chronic bronchitis patients with acute exacerbations [33]. We retrospectively analysed the results of a multicentre, double-blind, randomised, placebo-controlled trial carried out in 46 Italian general hospitals or university hospitals.

Patients were considered eligible if aged over 40 years with clinical diagnosis of chronic obstructive pulmonary disease defined by the presence of cough and sputum for at least 3 months in two consecutive years and forced expiratory volume in one second (FEV_1) below 80% of predicted value, determined in clinically stable conditions. Patients were excluded if they had reversible bronchial obstruction, malignancy, or severe hepatic, renal or cardiac failure. Patients receiving antibiotic or steroid therapy were also excluded. Seven hundred sixty-one eligible patients underwent a screening examination (between May and September 1989) during which past history data was recorded, focusing on the presence of exacerbations during the two previous winter seasons. Chest X-ray and lung function testing were performed.

The presence and severity of exacerbations were defined on the basis of the degree of severity of signs and symptoms measured by the semi-quantitative scales (Table 3). The sum of the six scores formed the exacerbation clinical score, which ranged from 0 to 18. Patients were considered eligible if at least one exacerbation had occurred in both the two previous years and basal clinical score was equal or below 8.

Eligible patients were followed as outpatients from October 1989 through April 1990. Patients were equipped with a diary for weekly recordings of any variation in breathlessness, sputum quantity and characteristics. Patients were instructed to phone or refer to our centre in case of critical variations of the parameters recorded in the diary. On such occasions patients would repeat all tests previously performed during the screening evaluation. Patients with pneumonia were excluded from the study.

The presence of exacerbation was established on the basis of critical variations in clinical scores compared to the screening score. Critical variation was defined as an increase of at least three points in the clinical score.

Table 3. Semi-quantitative scales defining the presence and severity of AECB (Modified from [33])

	Relative score			
	0	1	2	3
Cough	Absent	Mild[a]	Moderate[b]	Severe[c]
Body temperature (t)	$t \leq 37°\,C$	$37°\,C < t \leq 37.5°\,C$	$37.5°\,C < t \leq 38°\,C$	$t \leq 38°\,C$
Sputum quantity	Absent	Minimum (≤ 10 ml/day)	Moderate (≤ 15 ml/day)	Abundant (> 15 ml/day)
Sputum characteristics	Mucoid	Traces of purulence	$\leq 5\%$ purulence	$> 5\%$ purulence
Dyspnoea	Absent	Mild	Moderate	Severe
Pulmonary physical findings	Absent	Mild	Moderate	Severe

[a] Present on awakening and occasionally during the day.
[b] Present during most of the day.
[c] Causes disturbance to normal activities and nocturnal sleep.

Patients were randomised to one of the two treatment arms. Treatment was either amoxicillin-clavulanic acid (ratio 7:1) administered in 1 g tablets or placebo in indistinguishable tablets. The results of treatment were thus defined:

1. *Success*: reduction of clinical score to screening values;
2. *Improvement*: reduction of clinical score by at least two points;
3. *Failure*: reduction in clinical score by 1 point, no reduction or increase.

A follow-up examination and lung function testing were performed two weeks following symptom onset.

In our retrospective analysis of the 1991 data, we employed FEV_1 screening values, expressed as the percentage of predicted value, as the parameter for patient re-clustering on the basis of the degree of severity. Three clusters were identified: *Cluster 1* (104 patients), mean screening FEV_1 32.67 ± 6.83 (SD); *Cluster 2* (109 patients), mean screening FEV_1 54.12 ± 5.56; *Cluster 3* (122 patients), mean screening FEV_1 71.54 ± 5.51. The mean number of exacerbations during the 12 months prior to enrolment was 3.05 ± 0.96 and 1.61 ± 1.03 in Cluster 1 and Clusters 2+3, respectively ($p < 0.001$).

The success rate in the antibiotic group resulted significantly greater compared to the placebo group ($p < 0.001$). When clinical improvement was analysed on the basis of patient re-clustering, 16 of 51 Cluster 1 (severe COPD) patients treated with amoxicillin/clavulanate showed clinical improvement (31.4%), whereas success was recorded in 30 (58.8%). Conversely, among the 53 Cluster 1 patients receiving placebo, 7 (13.2%) improved and 9 (17%) successfully recovered ($p < 0.001$).

Mild and moderate COPD patients (Clusters 2 and 3) were grouped together. Among the 125 patients receiving antibiotic treatment in these 2 groups, 39 (31.2%) and 67 (53.6%) showed improvement or recovery, respectively, compared to 31 (29.2%) improvements and 32 (30.2%) successful recoveries among the 106 placebo-treated patients ($p < 0.001$).

The improvement/success vs. failure rate among amoxicillin/clavulanate treated patients in Cluster 1 subjects compared to Clusters 2+3 did not differ significantly. However, in placebo-treated patients the improvement/success vs. failure rate was significantly different in Cluster 1 patients compared to Clusters 2+3 subjects ($p < 0.01$).

The final FEV_1 values in the treatment and placebo groups were significantly different ($p < 0.01$) in favour of the active treatment group (Fig. 1). Among more severe patients (Cluster 1), the comparison between screening and follow-up FEV_1 values showed an improvement following antibiotic treatment and worsening after placebo. The difference between the two forms of treatment was highly significant ($p < 0.01$). Combining mild and moderate COPD patients (Clusters 2 and 3), the difference between screening and follow-up FEV_1 values was not significant for both treatment groups.

In summary, irrespective of disease severity, all clusters showed a significantly greater increase in the integrated clinical score following antibiotic treatment compared to placebo. In terms of lung function, our results show that the overall follow-up FEV_1 values were significantly greater among amoxicillin/clavulanate-treated patients than among placebo-treated patients. Furthermore, this difference showed the highest degree of significance among the cluster of more severe COPD patients.

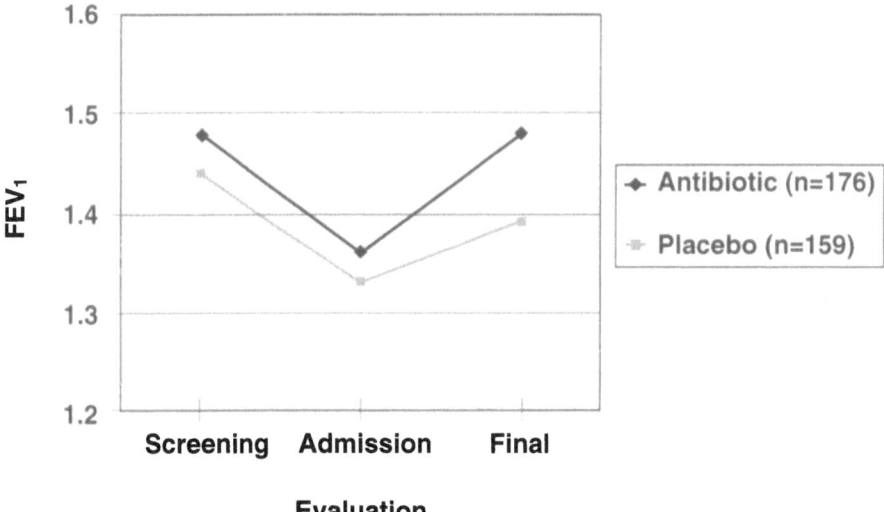

Fig. 1. FEV_1 values at screening, admission and final evaluation in patients with exacerbations of chronic bronchitis. Significant difference between antibiotic and placebo at final evaluation ($p < 0.01$) [33]

A significant finding is that among severe patients, placebo treatment was associated with worse clinical and functional outcomes compared to mild and moderately severe patients. This underscores the value of antibiotic treatment in patients with greater functional and clinical impairment (as determined by number of past exacerbations).

Conclusions

Exacerbations of chronic bronchitis are a common occurrence in clinical practice, and are a leading cause of antibiotic prescription among respiratory infections. It is still uncertain whether each new exacerbation may deteriorate the natural history of chronic bronchitis. Undoubtedly, every episode induces a temporary worsening in lung function and may therefore pose a threat of respiratory failure or death in more severely obstructed patients.

The overall impression from the studies performed on antibiotic value in AECB is that antibiotic treatment induces an improvement of both clinical and functional parameters. These benefits are in some studies relatively small but may be clinically significant, especially in patients with a more severe impairment of respiratory function.

In conclusion, the role of antibiotic treatment in chronic bronchitis exacerbations seems to be confirmed in terms of mid-term functional recovery, and to be relevant in patients with severe functional impairment and higher number of exacerbations per year in whom antibiotic treatment induces the greatest benefit.

References

1. Dantzker DR, Pingleton SK, Pierce JA, et al. (1987) Standards for the diagnosis and care of patients with chronic obstructive pulmonary disease and asthma. Am Rev Respir Dis 136:225-244
2. – (1994) Statistical abstract of the United States: 1994, 114th edn. US Bureau of the Census, Washington DC
3. Woolcock AJ (1989) Epidemiology of chronic airways disease. Chest 96(Suppl 3): 302S-306S
4. Murphy TF, Sethi S (1992) Bacterial infection in chronic obstructive pulmonary disease. Am Rev Respir Dis 146:1067-1083
5. Fagon JY, Chastre J, Trouillet JL, et al. (1990) Characterization of distal bronchial microflora during acute exacerbation of chronic bronchitis. Am Rev Respir Dis 142:1004-1008
6. Ball P (1995) Epidemiology and treatment of chronic bronchitis and its exacerbations. Chest 108(Suppl):43S-52S
7. Gump DW, Philips CA, Forsyth BR, McIntosh K, Lamborn KR, Stouch WH (1976) Role of infection in chronic bronchitis. Am Rev Respir Dis 113:465-474
8. Gump DW, Christmas WA, Forsyth BR, Philips CA, Stouch WH (1973) Serum and secretory antibodies in patients with chronic bronchitis. Arch Intern Med 132:847-851

9. Kanner RE, Renzetti AD Jr, Klauber MR, Smith CB, Golden CA (1979) Variables associated with spirometry in patients with obstructive lung disease. Am J Med 67:44-50
10. Cole P, Wilson R (1989) Host-microbial relationships in respiratory infection. Chest 95:217S-221S
11. Wilson R (1995) Outcome predictors in bronchitis. Chest 198(Suppl):53S-57S
12. Davies BL (1994) Critical review of microbiological data and methods in diagnosis of lower respiratory tract infections. Monaldi Arch Chest Dis 49:52-56
13. Ball P, Wilson R (1994) The epidemiology and management of chronic bronchits, the Cinderella of chest diseases. In: Ball AP, Wilson R (eds) Epidemiology and management of chronic bronchitis. Cambridge Medical, Worthing, pp III-IX
14. Blasi F, Legnani D, Lombardo VM, Negretto GG, Magliano E, Pozzoli R, Chiodo F, Fasoli A, Allegra L (1993) *Chlamydia pneumoniae* infection in acute exacerbations of COPD. Eur Respir J 6:19-22
15. The Working Party on Trials of Chemotherapy in Early Chronic Bronchitis of The Medical Research Council (1966) Value of chemoprophylaxis and chemotherapy in early chronic bronchitis. BMJ 1:317-322
16. Davis AL, Grobow EJ, Kaminski T, Tompsett R, McClement JH (1965) Bacterial infection and some effects of chemoprophylaxis in chronic pulmonary emphysema. II. Chemoprophylaxis with daily chloramphenicol. Am Rev Respir Dis 92:900-913
17. Priedie RB, Datta N, Massey DG, Poole GW, Schneeweiss J, Stradling P (1960) A trial of continuous winter chemotherapy in chronic bronchitis. Lancet 2:723-727
18. Francis RS, Spicer CC (1960) Chemotherapy in chronic bronchitis. Influence of daily penicillin and tetracycline on exacerbations and their costs. BMJ 1:297-303
19. Johnston RN, Lockart W, Smith DH, Cadman NK (1961) A trial of phenethicillin in chronic bronchitis. BMJ 2:985-986
20. Davis AL, Grobow EJ, Tompsett R, McClement JH (1961) Bacterial infection and some effects of chemoprophylaxis in chronic pulmonary emphysema. I. Chemoprophylaxis with intermittent tetracycline. Am J Med 31:365-381
21. Buchanan J, Buchanan WW, Melrose AG, McGuinness JB, Price AU (1958) Long-term prophylactic administration of tetracycline to chronic bronchitis. Lancet 2:719-722
22. Pines A (1967) Controlled trials of a sulphonamide given weekly to prevent exacerbations of chronic bronchitis. BMJ 3:202-204
23. Johnston RN, McNeill RS, Smith DH (1969) Five-year winter chemoprophylaxis for chronic bronchitis. BMJ 4:265-269
24. Murphy TF, Sethi S (1992) Bacterial infection in chronic obstructive pulmonary disease. Am Rev Respir Dis 146:1067-1083
25. Elmes PC, Fletcher CM, Dutton AAC (1957) Prophylactic use of oxytetracycline for exacerbations of chronic bronchitis. BMJ 2:1272-1275
26. Berry DG, Fry J, Hindley CP (1960) Exacerbations of chronic bronchitis treatment with oxytetracycline. Lancet 1:137-139
27. Fear EC, Edwards G (1962) Antibiotic regimens in chronic bronchitis. Br J Dis Chest 56:153-162
28. Elmes PC, King TKC, Langlands JHM (1965) Value of ampicillin in the hospital treatment of exacerbations of chronic bronchitis. BMJ 2:904-908
29. Petersen ES, Esmann V, Honke P, Munkner C (1967) A controlled study of the effect of treatment on chronic bronchitis: an evaluation using pulmonary function tests. Acta Med Scand 182:293-305
30. Pines A, Raafat H, Greenfield JSB, Linsell WD, Solari ME (1972) Antibiotic regimens in moderately ill patients with purulent exacerbations of chronic bronchitis. Br J Dis Chest 66:107-115

31. Nicotra MB, Rivera M, Awe RJ (1982) Antibiotic therapy of acute exacerbations of chronic bronchitis. Ann Intern Med 97:18-21
32. Anthonisen NR, Manfreda J, Warren CPW, Hershfield ES, Harding GKM, Nelson NA (1987) Antibiotic therapy in exacerbations of chronic obstructive pulmonary disease. Ann Intern Med 106:196-204
33. Allegra L, Grassi C, Grossi E, Pozzi E, Blasi F, Frigerio D, Nastri A, Montanari C, Montanari M, Serra G (1991) Ruolo degli antibiotici nel trattamento delle riacutizzazioni della bronchite cronica: risultati di uno studio italiano multicentrico. Ital J Chest Dis 45:138-148
34. Jorgensen AF, Coolidge J, Pedersen PA (1992) Amoxicillin in treatment of acute uncomplicated exacerbations of chronic bronchitis. Scand J Prim Health Care 10:7-11
35. Saint S, Bent S, Vittinghoff E, Grady D (1995) Antibiotics in chronic obstructive pulmonary disease exacerbations. A meta-analysis. JAMA 273(12):957-960
36. Eller J, Ede A, Schaberg T, Niederman MS, Mauch H, Lode H (1998) Infective exacerbations of chronic bronchitis. Relation between bacteriologic etiology and lung function. Chest 113:1542-1548
37. Huchon G, Woodhead M (1998) Management of adult community-acquired lower respiratory tract infections. Eur Respir Rev 8:391-426
38. Dewan N, Destache CJ, O'Donohue WJ Jr, Campbell JC, Angelillo VA (1994) Antibiotic choice and office visits for acute exacerbation of chronic bronchitis. Chest 106(Suppl):161S

Infection and Antibiotic Treatment in Acute Exacerbations of Chronic Bronchitis

M.S. Niederman

Introduction

Patients with chronic bronchitis commonly have disease exacerbations, characterized by any or all of three "cardinal symptoms": increased dyspnea, increased sputum volume and increased sputum purulence. In one study, Anthonisen and colleagues graded exacerbations as type I if all three symptoms were present, type II if only two symptoms were present, and type III if only one symptom was present [1]. Although bacterial infection may be responsible for exacerbations, and antibiotics are commonly prescribed, this type of therapy remains controversial, particularly since only half of all exacerbations are bacterial in origin, the rest being viral or chemical. Thus, some believe that antibiotic therapy of acute exacerbations of chronic bronchitis (AECB) is an abuse of antibiotics, and can contribute to antimicrobial resistance. However, a recent meta-analysis has concluded that antibiotics are of benefit, and available data show that this benefit is most clear in patients who have at least two of the three cardinal symptoms of exacerbation [2].

The other controversial aspect of antibiotic therapy of AECB is whether it matters which antibiotic is used. For example, in the American Thoracic Society (ATS) guidelines for chronic obstructive pulmonary disease (COPD), any antibiotic is considered likely to be effective, and thus it makes no difference which one is chosen [3]. In spite of this view, guidelines for the therapy of AECB have been published, and they take the approach that there are differences in the bacteriology of exacerbation in different patient populations, defining patient subsets that require different therapies [4]. The concept of patient subsets among those with chronic bronchitis is now beginning to be validated, but the impact of using subsets for antibiotic selection is less certain. Still, when antibiotics are used according to guidelines, there is the implicit concept that the benefits of antibiotics may be dramatic for individuals with severe acute

Pulmonary and Critical Care Division and Department of Medicine, Winthrop-University Hospital, Mineola, NY, USA; Department of Medicine, State University of New York at Stony Brook, Stony Brook, NY, USA and chronic illness, while the impact of no therapy, or failed therapy, may be catastrophic, leading to hospitalization and even mechanical ventilation.

Thus, many questions and controversies remain when considering antibiotic therapy for AECB, and these are discussed below.

Do Antibiotics Have a Benefit in AECB?

Patients with COPD have on average 3 exacerbations per year, with one-third of all patients having < 3 episodes, one-third having 3 episodes, and one-third having 4 or more episodes [5]. Most exacerbations are managed out of the hospital, and one recent study examined the epidemiology and cost of AECB in the United States, acknowledging that it was difficult to measure the number of outpatients treated annually [6]. Using 1994 data, the authors estimated that there were 280 000 admissions for AECB and over 10 million outpatient visits (and maybe many more) for this illness. For the admitted patients, those age 65 years or older accounted for 207 540 admissions, while those < age 65 years accounted for 73 299 admissions. The older patients had a mean length of stay of 6.3 days for a total cost of US \$1.1 billion, while the younger patients had a mean length of stay of 5.8 days for a total cost of US \$419 million. For the outpatients, 5.8 million episodes were in those age 65 years or older, while 4.2 million episodes were in the younger population. When care was given out of the hospital, for those treated in an office, emergency room, or hospital clinic, the cost of an exacerbation was between \$74 and \$159 per episode [6]. In contrast, for an inpatient, the average cost was \$5516 per episode. In both outpatient and inpatient settings, antibiotics made up a small amount of total cost, accounting for 15% and 11%, respectively, of all costs. The data in this study make it clear that the major cost increment in this illness comes with hospital admission, and thus if an antibiotic is used during exacerbation and can prevent hospitalization, it will be a highly cost-effective therapy.

One of the reasons that antibiotic therapy of AECB is controversial is that the same bacteria can be found in the sputum of patients when they are healthy and when they are ill, since most COPD patient have chronic airway colonization. The most commonly recovered organisms are non-typable *Haemophilus influenzae*, pneumococcus, and *Moraxella catarrhalis*. Although the role of these bacteria in exacerbations is uncertain, most experts agree that up to half of all exacerbations are bacterial in origin [7, 8]. In addition, bacterial pathogens could play several other important roles: they could serve as secondary infecting agents after viral or chemical tracheobronchitis [9]; or they could contribute to progressive airway destruction through the induction of a host inflammatory response and by the production of inflammatory exoproducts, both of which could lead to airway injury as a byproduct of inflammation [10]. This last role occurs through a "vicious cycle" of lung inflammation and injury leading to bacterial colonization which in turn creates more airway inflammation and injury, more bacterial infection, and an associated loss of lung function. If such a vicious cycle is operating in patients with COPD, then periodic courses of antibiotics could break this cycle and slow the progression of airway obstruction. However, only one of four prospective studies has shown that a more rapid decline in lung function occurs in patients with more frequent exacerbations [11].

While some of the benefits of antibiotics are theoretical, their real value comes from data collected in prospective, randomized, placebo-controlled trials that have shown some benefit during acute exacerbations, but no benefit if used to prevent exacerbations [2, 11]. One recent meta-analysis evaluated nine randomized and placebo-controlled trials of antibiotic therapy in AECB, conducted between 1957 and 1992 [2]; this analysis showed a small beneficial effect of antibiotic therapy when the endpoints were overall benefit and change in peak flow rate. Another analysis of placebo-controlled trials for AECB, conducted by Ball, reached similar conclusions [12].

Probably the best single study of AECB was that of Anthonisen and colleagues, reported in 1987 from Canada, involving a total of 362 exacerbations in 173 patients studied in a placebo-controlled, randomized, double-blinded study design [1]. Patients who received antibiotic therapy were treated for 10 days with either trimethoprim-sulfamethoxazole, amoxicillin, or doxycycline out of a belief that these antibiotics could be used interchangeably since they were thought to be equally effective. This assumption may not currently be correct, because of our understanding of differences among patients, and because of an increased frequency of antibiotic resistance present now, compared to the early 1980s. In the study, each exacerbation was graded according to the number of cardinal symptoms present: nearly 40% of all exacerbations were the most severe (type I), with all three cardinal symptoms present; 40% were type II; and 20% were type III, with only one symptom present. Antibiotic-treated patients did significantly better than placebo-treated patients, showing a more rapid return of peak flow, a greater percentage of patients showing clinical success, and a smaller percentage showing clinical failure. However, the benefits were most evident in patients with at least two cardinal symptoms present: the 80% of individuals with type I or type II exacerbations. The data in this study were confirmed in an Italian study that defined severity of acute exacerbation by accounting for symptoms of cough and the presence of concomitant illness [13].

The data from Anthonisen, et al.'s study suggest that antibiotics should be given to patients who have at least two of the three cardinal symptoms. This approach is preferred to one of trying to distinguish a bacterial from a nonbacterial (chemical or viral) exacerbation, particularly since clinical features cannot reliably distinguish between these two possibilities. In one study of 54 patients with severe episodes (requiring mechanical ventilation) of bronchial infection complicating COPD, 27 patients had bacteria recovered from the airway using a protected specimen brush sampling technique [8]. When patients with secretions containing bacteria were compared to those with sterile secretions, there were no differences with regard to duration of symptoms, fever, white blood cell count, or degree of hypoxemia.

Although the data show that antibiotics lead to more rapid and more frequent resolution of AECB than does placebo treatment, there are several additional potential benefits of antibiotic therapy for patients with chronic bronchitis (Table 1). For example, antibiotics could reduce the burden of bacteria in the airway. Since many exacerbations involve high concentrations of bacteria, the

Table 1. Potential benefits of antibiotic therapy for acute exacerbations of chronic bronchitis

Immediate, short-term benefits
    Reduce the duration of symptoms, lead to a more rapid return of peak flow rates, with associated clinical cure and a lower likelihood of clinical deterioration
        Prevent hospitalization
        Facilitate an earlier return to work
    Prevent progression to pneumonia from severe tracheobronchial infection

Long-term benefits
    Prevent loss of lung function by breaking the vicious cycle of infection and airway injury
    Prolong the disease-free interval between exacerbations
    Prevent secondary bacterial infection after documented viral infection

reduction in counts brought about by therapy might be able to prevent some episodes of bronchitis from progressing to pneumonia. A study comparing sputum samples using Gram's stain showed that patients with AECB had 8-18 organisms per oil immersion field, compared to fewer than 2 organisms per field for stable patients [14]. Similarly, bronchoscopy studies of this illness have shown that as many as 52%-72% of outpatients or inpatients with AECB have bacteria present, often at concentrations $> 10^3$ organisms/ml in a protected specimen brush (PSB) sample [8, 14-16]. Since a concentration of $> 10^3$ organisms/ml PSB sample has been used to define the presence of pneumonia in hospitalized patients with lung infiltrates, many patients with AECB have as many bacteria in their airway as if they had pneumonia. If antibiotics can reduce this bacterial burden, some AECB patients will be prevented from progressing from airway infection to parenchymal lung infection. In addition, even viral exacerbations are sometimes complicated by secondary bacterial infections [9]. These events may be avoided by antibiotic therapy, demonstrating another benefit of the relatively routine use of these agents.

What Organisms Should Be Targeted in AECB Therapy? How Commonly Are They Antibiotic-Resistant?

The three most common organisms causing acute exacerbations of chronic bronchitis are *H. influenzae*, pneumococcus, and *M. catarrhalis*. The frequency of these organisms and the likelihood that they are antibiotic resistant vary with the profile of risk factors present in a given patient. In outpatients with exacerbations of mild severity, *H. influenzae* predominates, followed by the other organisms (pneumococcus and *M. catarrhalis*); gram-negative infection is relatively uncommon [15]. In patients with severe exacerbations, *H. influenzae* is less common and *H. parainfluenzae* is the most common organism isolated from bronchoscopy samples; gram-negative bacteria are also frequently isolated [8].

Haemophilus influenzae, usually non-encapsulated and thus non-typable, is the most common organism leading to exacerbation. It produces beta-lacta-mase which digests and destroys traditional beta-lactam antibiotics such as ampicillin or amoxicillin. In one study, as many as 40% of *H. influenzae* strains produced this enzyme, and some produced so much that they were resistant to amoxicillin-clavulanate [17]. In addition, 2.5% of these clinical isolates were beta-lactamase negative yet ampicillin resistant, due to the presence of altered penicillin-binding proteins [17]. Beta-lactamase production is even more common with *Moraxella catarrhalis*, and one study found these enzymes in 95% of 723 isolates [18].

Pneumococcal resistance to common antibiotics is increasingly frequent, being present in as many as 40% of all isolates, although much of this resistance is intermediate and not high-level resistance; thus the implications of resistance for antibiotic therapy are uncertain [19]. Resistance is more likely if patients have identified risk factors such as: age > 65 years, alcoholism, beta-lactam therapy within the previous 3 months, multiple medical comorbidities, and immune-suppressive illness [19, 20].

How Can We Define Patient Subsets for Therapy?

Patients can be divided into different categories, with different subsets being at risk for specific pathogens. In order to characterize patients, it is necessary to define age (< or ≥ 65 years), frequency of exacerbations, presence of comorbid cardiopulmonary disease, frequency of antibiotic therapy, use of cortico-steroids, and severity of obstructive airway disease (FEV_1 as a percentage are of predicted). All patients are at risk for the three core organisms, namely *H. influenzae*, pneumococcus, and *M. catarrhalis*. As patients become increasingly complex, the likelihood of antibiotic resistance among these organisms increases, as does the frequency of the more difficult to treat gram-negative organisms.

Bronchoscopic studies have shown that as the severity of exacerbation increases, the bacteriology of the exacerbation changes. While stable outpatients usually are infected with the core organisms, those requiring mechanical ventilation for AECB have an increased frequency of gram-negative organisms [8, 15, 16]. In addition, two recent studies have related the bacteriology of exacerbations to the severity of baseline lung function, as defined by FEV_1 as a percentage of predicted normal [21, 22]. In one study of 112 COPD patients, lung function fell into three stages: FEV_1 ≥ 50% of predicted, FEV_1 36%-49% of predicted, and FEV_1 ≤ 35% of predicted. Bacteria were also categorized into three groups: pneumococcus and other gram positives, *H. influenzae* and *M. catarrhalis*, and gram negatives including *Enterobacteriaceae* and *P. aeruginosa*. Although the enteric gram negatives were more common than any other class of bacteria during AECB, these organisms were most common in patients with the most severe lung dysfunction, while the gram positives predominated in the exacerbations of patients with the mildest degree of lung function abnormalities. Similarly, in another study of 148 ambulatory patients with type I or type II exacerbations, those with an FEV_1 < 50% of predicted were more likely to have *H. influenzae* and *P. aeruginosa* than patients with better lung function [22].

Other studies have identified the frequency of exacerbations and the presence of comorbid cardiopulmonary disease as factors to be considered in defining patient subsets. In one study of 471 outpatients with AECB, the likelihood of a patient having a recurrence after therapy for exacerbation was related to these factors [5]. If patients had < 3 exacerbations per year, then the recurrence rate was 9.1%, compared to 13.1% in those with 3-4 exacerbations per year, and 18.4% in those with > 4 exacerbations per year. A factor such as age is important in defining patient subsets because age > 65 years has been identified as a risk factor for airway colonization by gram negatives, and for antibiotic resistance if pneumococcus is present [19, 20].

The definition of patient subsets should be considered for the selection of antibiotics for two reasons. First, different subsets of patients are at risk for infection with different organisms. Second, those in the more complex categories may have a greater "cost of failure" of empiric therapy than less complex patients.

What Are the Characteristics of the "Ideal Antibiotic" for AECB?

Studies of AECB therapy generally do not show clear superiority of one agent over another, because most often they are designed to show equivalence between a new agent and a previously approved agent. In addition, the use of patient subsets to choose therapy has not been formally tested in a prospective fashion. However, some principles are logical in the selection of antibiotics for AECB (Table 2) and these require that the chosen agent have certain features, as follows.

Table 2. Characteristics of the ideal antibiotic for AECB

Active against the core organisms (pneumococcus, *H. influenzae, M. catarrhalis*) and possibly against atypical pathogens

Active against enteric gram negatives and resistant pathogens in selected patients

Resistant to destruction by bacterial beta-lactamases (produced by *H. influenzae, M. catarrhalis*)

Good penetration into sputum and bronchial tissue: high sputum/MIC ratio against target organisms

Good likelihood of compliance with therapy: once- or twice-daily dosing, few side effects

Cost-effective, especially regarding prevention of hospitalization and prolongation of time between exacerbations

Antimicrobial Activity

The agents most commonly used to treat patients with AECB include: beta-lactams (penicillins and cephalosporins), macrolides and azalides (erythromycin, clarithromycin and azithromycin), tetracyclines, trimethoprim-sulfamethoxazole and quinolones.

Macrolides and Tetracyclines

Macrolides are bacteriostatic agents that bind to the 50S ribosomal subunit of the target bacteria and inhibit RNA-dependent protein synthesis. They have good activity against pneumococci, as well as against atypical pathogens (*C. pneumoniae, M. pneumoniae, Legionella*). However, the older erythromycin-type drugs are not active against *H. influenzae*, interact with theophylline to increase its levels, and have poor intestinal tolerance, making it difficult to use these agents in patients with AECB. The new macrolide agents, including azithromycin (an azalide) and clarithromycin, have enhanced activity against *H. influenzae* (including beta-lactamase-producing strains); nonetheless, on the basis of minimum inhibitory concentration (MIC), azithromycin is more active [23, 24]. The macrolides are also active against *M. catarrhalis*, although the new agents have enhanced activity against this pathogen, compared to the older agents. Among the new macrolides, azithromycin is more active than erythromycin against not only *H. influenzae* and *M. catarrhalis*, but also *M. pneumoniae*. On the other hand, clarithromycin is more active against *S. pneumoniae, Legionella* and *C. pneumoniae* [23, 24]. Azithromycin has no theophylline interaction, while clarithromycin has the same potential for interaction as does erythromycin.

Both of the newer agents have better intestinal tolerance than erythromycin and penetrate well into sputum, lung tissue and phagocytes. Clarithromycin, which has an active 14-hydroxy metabolite that is antibacterial, is administered twice a day orally at a 500 mg dose for 10 days in the treatment of community-acquired pneumonia (CAP). Azithromycin has a longer half-life than clarithromycin and concentrates in tissues, achieving very low serum levels when administered orally. The dose for oral therapy of AECB is 500 mg on day one, followed by 250 mg daily on days 2-5.

Macrolides remain an important therapeutic option for AECB, but one concern is that pneumococci are becoming increasingly resistant to macrolides, particularly in conjunction with penicillin resistance. In one study, 30%-40% of all the pneumococci that were intermediate or high-level penicillin resistant were also erythromycin resistant [19]. The clinical relevance of these in vitro findings remains to be defined. However, there are two forms of macrolide resistance, one involving efflux of the antibiotic from the bacterial cell, and the other involving altered ribosomal binding of the antibiotic. The former mechanism is associated with much lower levels of resistance than the latter. If the latter form of resistance is present, then it is unlikely that macrolide therapy for pneumococcal infection would be effective.

The tetracyclines are also bacteriostatic agents that act by binding the 30S ribosomal subunit and interfering with protein synthesis. These agents can be used in AECB because they are active against *H. influenzae* and atypical pathogens, but there are reports of increasing resistance among pneumococci [23, 24]. Photosensitivity is the major side effect, limiting the use of these agents in sun-exposed patients.

Trimethoprim-Sulfamethoxazole

This combination antibiotic has been used as a mainstay for the therapy of AECB because of its antimicrobial spectrum, ease of use, and low cost. Trimethoprim-sulfamethoxazole (TMP-SMX) is bactericidal against pneumococcus, *H. influenzae* and *M. catarrhalis*, but not atypical pathogens. TMP-SMX is administered both orally and intravenously in a fixed combination of 1:5 (TMP:SMX), and dosage should be adjusted in renal failure. Side effects generally result from the sulfamethoxazole component and include rash, gastrointestinal (GI) upset and, occasionally, renal failure. The major limitation to using this agent in AECB relates to increasing rates of resistance among a variety of organisms including pneumococcus. If a pneumococcal organism is penicillin-resistant, then it has an 80%-90% likelihood of also being resistant to TMP-SMX [19].

Beta-Lactam Antibiotics

These bactericidal antibiotics, which include the penicillins, cephalosporins and other agents, have in common the presence of a beta-lactam ring, which is bound to a five-membered thiazolidine ring in the penicillins and to a six-membered dihydrothiazine ring in the cephalosporins [23, 24]. Beta-lactam antibiotics work by interfering with the synthesis of bacterial cell wall peptidoglycans by binding to bacterial penicillin-binding proteins. These agents can also be combined with beta-lactamase inhibitors such as sulbactam, tazobactam or clavulanic acid to create the beta-lactam/beta-lactamase inhibitor drugs. These compounds extend the antimicrobial spectrum of the beta-lactams by providing a substrate for the bacterial beta-lactamases (sulbactam, clavulanic acid, tazobactam).

The penicillins used for AECB include the aminopenicillins (ampicillin, amoxicillin) and the beta-lactam/beta-lactamase inhibitor combinations. The antipseudomonal penicillins are administered only intravenously, and are not commonly used for AECB. The beta-lactamase inhibitor combination most commonly used for oral therapy of AECB is amoxicillin-clavulanate. Nonetheless as discussed previously, some *H. influenzae* strains over-produce beta-lactamase enzymes enough to be resistant to amoxicillin-clavulanate [17].

The cephalosporins span from first to fourth generations. The earlier agents were generally active against gram positives, but did not have extended activity to the more complex gram negatives, or anaerobes, and were susceptible to destruction by bacterial beta-lactamases. The newer generation agents are generally more specialized, with broad spectrum activity, and with more mechanisms to resist breakdown by bacteria. The second generation and newer agents are resistant to bacterial beta-lactamases, and the oral agents that are active against resistant pneumococci include cefuroxime, cefprozil, and cefpodoxime. The intravenous third and fourth generation agents active against penicillin-resistant pneumococci include ceftriaxone, cefotaxime, and cefepime, while ceftazidime is less reliable against this organism.

Fluoroquinolones

These bactericidal agents act by interfering with bacterial DNA gyrase, leading to impaired DNA synthesis repair, transcription and other cellular processes, resulting in bacterial cell lysis [25]. DNA gyrase is one form of bacterial topo-isomerases that are inhibited by quinolones, but activity against other similar enzymes is part of the effect of a variety of quinolones. Quinolones kill bacteria in a concentration-dependent fashion: the higher the concentration of the antibiotic relative to the MIC of the target organism, the more rapidly the bacteria is killed and the lower the chance to develop resistance. This activity can be expressed as the ratio of the peak serum concentration to MIC (Cmax/MIC ratio) or as the ratio of the area under the concentration-time curve to the MIC (AUC/MIC ratio). In the therapy of CAP, the optimal Cmax/MIC ratio for a quinolone is between 10:1 and 12:1 [26].

There are two features of quinolones which make them suited to respiratory infections. First, they penetrate well into respiratory secretions and inflammatory cells, achieving concentrations that usually exceed serum levels. Thus, these agents may be clinically more effective than predicted by MIC values. This may explain the observation that quinolones are often better than other agents in prolonging the "disease-free" interval between exacerbations [7]. Second, these agents are highly bioavailable with oral administration and thus similar levels can be reached if administered orally or intravenously.

The fluoroquinolones are highly active against beta-lactamase-producing *H. influenzae* and *M. catarrhalis*, making them very useful for patients with AECB. Currently, a number of new quinolones has become available, which extend the activity of the older agents by providing enhanced gram-positive activity; they are also more active against *C. pneumoniae* and *M. pneumoniae* than the older agents [25]. The new agents are also highly effective against *L. pneumophila*. However, if *P. aeruginosa* is the target organism, then only ciprofloxacin and trovafloxacin (which is not being used because of toxicity issues) are active enough for clinical use. One of the problems with the older agents, ciprofloxacin and ofloxacin, was their borderline activity against pneumococcus. Thus, when these agents have been used for AECB, optimal success was achieved with high doses. For example, one recent study showed that ciprofloxacin was effective for the therapy of complex patients with AECB, but the dose used was 750 mg twice daily [27].

A variety of newer agents has become available, with enhanced gram-positive activity, yet with preserved antimicrobial effects against the other common AECB pathogens. These agents include (in order of increasing activity against pneumococcus): levofloxacin, sparfloxacin, grepafloxacin, trovafloxacin, gatifloxacin, moxifloxacin, and gemifloxacin [28] (Table 3). One recent study has

Table 3. Serum activity of fluoroquinolones against pneumococcus

Agent (dosage)	MIC 90 (mg/l)	Serum Cmax (mg/l)
Grepafloxacin (400 mg)	0.25-0.5	1.4
Levofloxacin (500 mg)[a]	1.0	5.7
Sparfloxacin (200 mg)	0.25-0.5	1.4
Trovafloxacin (200 mg)	0.125-0.25	3.1
Gatifloxacin (400 mg)	0.5	3.8
Moxifloxacin (400 mg)[a]	0.25	4.5
Ciprofloxacin (500 mg)	2.0	2.4
Gemifloxacin (320 mg)	0.015	1.2

[a] Not highly protein-bound, leading to high free concentrations; clinical relevance is unknown; *MIC*, minimum inhibitory concentration

shown that as organisms become penicillin resistant, they are also more likely to be quinolone resistant [28]. With this in mind, pneumococci are less likely to be resistant to the agents with the best pneumococcal activity, and thus the differences between agents may become clinically relevant in the immediate future. These new agents also have long half-lives, generally allowing for once-daily dosing: the half-lives of these drugs vary from as short as 6 h for levofloxacin to as long as > 15 h for moxifloxacin and grepafloxacin. One major distinction among these new quinolones is their profile of toxic side effects, which along with efficacy, must be considered when choosing a specific agent.

Antibiotic Penetration into the Lung

To assure the optimal effect of an antibiotic, it is necessary that the drug reach the site of infection, the bronchial mucosa. Antibiotics can concentrate in a variety of sites in the lung, including the sputum, the bronchial epithelium, the lung parenchyma, the epithelial lining fluid and phagocytic cells [29]. Although it is unclear which site is most relevant in AECB therapy, concentrations in the mucosa and sputum seem most relevant. Drugs which are lipid-soluble penetrate well into sputum and bronchial mucosa, regardless of the presence of inflammation, and include the macrolides, tetracycline, quinolones and trimethoprim-sulfamethoxazole. Another way to express the local concentration of an antibiotic for bronchial infection is to compare the achieved sputum level to the MIC of the target organism. When a quinolone such as ciprofloxacin is used, the sputum to MIC ratio for *H. influenzae* and *M. catarrhalis* exceeds a value of 60. The macrolide azithromycin has a sputum/MIC ratio for pneumococcus that exceeds 60 as well. Although the ratio for the newer macrolides against *H. influenzae* is considerably lower, the ratio for clarithromycin against pneumococcus exceeds a value of 250 [30]. The clinical relevance of these findings for therapeutic efficacy remains uncertain.

Ease of Use

Patient compliance is essential in the therapy of AECB, but studies have shown that compliance with short-term antibiotic regimens ranges anywhere from 56% to 89% [31]. Patients are less likely to comply with a prescribed regimen if they are already taking multiple medications, if side effects occur, if dosing is more than twice a day, if use conflicts with their lifestyle, and if the consequences of non-compliance seem minimal. In a recent survey, 54% of all Americans reported that they did not finish a course of antibiotics as prescribed, and many stopped antibiotics once they felt better, even if they had not finished a full course of therapy [32]. When questioned, 82% of the respondents preferred an antibiotic that can be given once or twice a day, and only 5% were willing to be treated for a 14-day course [32].

With this in mind, a number of appropriate antibiotics for AECB can be given once or twice a day. Once-daily dosing is possible with azithromycin and the new quinolones. Other oral antibiotics are also available for once-daily dosing, but do not represent ideal drugs from an antimicriobial spectrum; these include cefixime, ceftibutin, and dirithromycin. Twice-daily dosing is feasible with amoxicillin-clavulanate, cefpodoxime, cefuroxime, ciprofloxacin, clarithromycin, doxycycline, ofloxacin and trimethoprim-sulfamethoxazole.

Cost-effectiveness

Although it is difficult to define the cost-effectiveness of antibiotic therapy, it is quite clear that if an agent costs little to buy but has limited efficacy, it might cause a patient to miss several days of work. Therefore, such an agent is less cost-effective than a more expensive agent able to cure the patient rapidly. Other endpoints to be considered in defining a cost-effective antibiotic for AECB include the prevention of hospitalization, the duration of disease-free intervals, the need for other medications, and the development of antimicrobial resistance.

One recent study illustrated the value of accurate antibiotic choices, even if the acquisition cost is higher than that of less accurate antibiotic strategies [33]. A total of 224 exacerbations in 60 outpatients was examined, and therapy was based on first-line (amoxicillin, tetracycline, erythromycin, trimethoprim-sulfamethoxazole), second-line (cephalosporins) or third-line (amoxicillin-clavulanate, azithromycin, ciprofloxacin) agents. Patients who received third-line agents failed less often than those who received first-line agents (7% vs. 19%, $p < 0.05$) [33]. In addition, those given third-line agents were hospitalized less often than those with first-line agents, and the time between exacerbations was significantly longer for those using third-line agents. Another study, using a pharmacoeconomic model to evaluate 1102 patients with AECB in previously reported randomized trials, concluded that macrolide therapy and therapy with amoxicillin-clavulanate were more cost-effective than therapy with ampicillin and older cephalosporins [34].

One other study looking at this issue was a prospective randomized trial of quinolone therapy (with ciprofloxacin) versus usual care, involving 240 patients with AECB managed by their family physicians [35]. For the group as a whole, quinolone therapy was not substantially better than usual care, but for certain patient subsets it appeared to have some advantage. Ciprofloxacin was associated with a better clinical outcome and lower costs for patients who had moderate or severe bronchitis (severity of the acute episode), at least 4 episodes of AECB in the preceding year, > 10 years illness, age 56 years or greater, and at least 3 comorbidities, once again confirming the concept that empiric therapy should be modified for different patient groups. These findings suggest that if patient profiling is used to prescribe antibiotics, then the benefits of therapy with selected agents for specific patients will be enhanced.

Guidelines for Therapy of AECB Using Patient Subsets

Patients with AECB can be classified into one of three groups: (1) uncomplicated AECB, (2) complicated AECB, and (3) AECB at risk for *P. aeruginosa* and other resistant gram-negative pathogens. This stratification is based on the previously discussed risk factors and considers that certain patients are at risk for specific organisms, while others are not. In addition, the stratification assumes that patients with more severe acute and chronic illness, particularly those at risk for drug-resistant organisms, need an aggressive approach to initial antibiotic therapy, since the "cost of failure" of such therapy may be great in both medical and economic terms. The following guidelines discuss each of the three AECB patient groups and the individual recommended therapies (Table 4).

Therapy for all patients should target the group of core organisms that includes *H. influenzae* (usually non-typable), *M. catarrhalis* and *S. pneumoniae*. Patients at risk for only these organisms fall into the uncomplicated AECB group. This group includes patients of any age having < 4 exacerbations/year, no comorbid illness, and an FEV_1 > 50% of predicted. This type of patient can be treated with first-line antibiotics, provided that there are at least two of the

Table 4. Proposed therapies for AECB, according to patient subsets

Patient group	Therapy options for type I or type II exacerbations
Uncomplicated AECB	Macrolides (azithromycin, clarithromycin), New cephalosporins (cefpodoxime, cefuroxime, cefprozil), Doycycline
Complicated AECB	Fluoroquinolones Amoxicillin-clavulanate
AECB at risk for *P. aeruginosa*	Quinolone with anti-pseudomonal activity (ciprofloxacin)

three cardinal symptoms of an exacerbation. The first-line antibiotics do not necessarily cover resistant organisms and enteric gram-negatives since these are unlikely in an uncomplicated patient. First-line agents include the newer macrolides (azithromycin or clarithromycin), the cephalosporins (cefuroxime, cefpodoxime, cefprozil), or doxycycline. Although ampicillin, amoxicillin and the first-generation cephalosporins could be used in this setting, their suscepti-bility to the increasingly common bacterial beta-lactamases limits their utility. Trimethoprim-sulfamethoxazole is of limited value because of increasing rates of pneumococcal resistance and because of side effects. Erythromycin is of lim-ited value because of side effects and insufficient activity against *H. influenzae.*

The complicated AECB patient is one who is generally older than age 65 years and has more than 4 exacerbations per year, serious comorbid illness or an FEV_1 < 50% of predicted. This patient is at risk for the core organisms, but also is more likely to have drug-resistant organisms (beta-lactamase-producing organisms, and resistant pneumococcus), and possibly enteric gram-negative bacteria. Recommended therapy for this population is oral fluoroquinolone with enhanced pneumococcal activity, or alternatively amoxicillin-clavulanate. One advantage of quinolone in this setting is the excellent penetration to the bronchial mucosa and sputum, achieving higher levels, relative to serum con-centrations, than beta-lactam antibiotics.

The patient at risk for *P. aeruginosa* is the most difficult to effectively treat. These patients are defined as those with: chronic bronchial sepsis; need for chron-ic corticosteroid therapy and frequent courses of antibiotics (> 4 times per year); or an FEV_1 < 35% of predicted. These patients should be treated with ciprofloxacin, the only currently available oral agent that is active against *P. aerug-inosa.*

This stratification scheme must be viewed as a hypothesis to be verified with prospectively collected data. Such studies can document whether patient outcome is improved when this scheme is followed. However, as previously dis-cussed, preliminary studies do support the general approach in these recom-mendations. More data are needed to define the optimal duration of therapy for an acute exacerbation of AECB, although many trials have shown efficacy with a 5- to 7-day course in uncomplicated patients. In more severely ill patients with more complex disease, the duration of therapy should be determined by the rate of symptom resolution, and 10-14 days of antibiotics may be needed to avoid relapse. In addition, future studies must examine the time between exa-cerbations as an important endpoint and should define whether the use of patient stratification to guide therapy can impact on this outcome.

References

1. Anthonisen NR, Manfreda J, Warren CPW, et al. (1987) Antibiotic therapy in exacer-bations of chronic obstructive pulmonary disease. Ann Intern Med 106:196-204
2. Saint S, Bent S, Vittinghoff E, Grady D (1995) Antibiotics in chronic obstructive pulmonary disease exacerbations: A meta-analysis. JAMA 273:957-960

3. American Thoracic Society (1995) Standards for the diagnosis and care of patients with chronic obstructive pulmonary disease. Am J Respir Crit Care Med 152:S77-S120

4. Balter MS, Hyland RH, Low DE, Renzi PM, et al. (1994) Recommendations on the management of chronic bronchitis: A practical guide for Canadian physicians. Can Med Assoc J 151(10)(Suppl):5-23

5. Ball P, Harris JM, Lowson D, et al. (1995) Acute infective exacerbations of chronic bronchitis. Q J Med 88:61-68

6. Niederman MS, McCombs JS, Unger AN, Kumar A, Popovian R (1999) Treatment cost of acute exacerbations of chronic bronchitis. Clin Ther 21:576-591

7. Chodosh S (1991) Treatment of chronic bronchitis: state of the art. Am J Med 91(6A):87S-92S

8. Fagon JY, Chastre J, Trouillet JL, et al. (1990) Characterization of distal bronchial microflora during acute exacerbation of chronic bronchitis: Use of the protected specimen brush technique in 54 mechanically ventilated patients. Am Rev Respir Dis 142:1004-1008

9. Smith CB, Golden C, Klauber MR, et al. (1976) Interaction between viruses and bacteria in patients with chronic bronchitis. J Infect Dis 134: 552-561

10. Wilson R (1995) Outcome predictors in bronchitis. Chest 108:53S-57S

11. Murphy TF, Sethi S (1992) Bacterial infection in chronic obstructive pulmonary disease. Am Rev Respir Dis 146:1067-1083

12. Ball P (1995) Epidemiology and treatment of chronic bronchitis and its exacerbations. Chest 108:43S-52S

13. Allegra L, Grassi C, Grossi, et al. (1991) Ruolo degli antibiotici nel trattamento delle riacutizza della bronchite cronica. Ital J Chest Dis 45:38-48

14. Baigelman W, Chodosh S, Pizzuto D, et al. (1979) Quantitative sputum Gram stains in chronic bronchial disease. Lung 156:265-270

15. Monso E, Ruiz J, Rosell A, et al. (1995) Bacterial infection in chronic obstructive pulmonary disease: A study of stable and exacerbated outpatients using the protected specimen brush. Am J Respir Crit Care Med 152:1316-1320

16. Soler N, Torres A, Ewig S, Gonzalez J, Celis R, El-Ebiary M, et al. (1998) Bronchial microbial patterns in severe exacerbations of chronic obstructive pulmonary disease (COPD) requiring mechanical ventilation. Am J Respir Crit Care Med 157:1498-1505

17. Doern GV, Brueggemann AB, Pierce G, Holley HP Jr, Rauch A (1997) Antibiotic resistance among clinical isolates of *Haemophilus influenzae* in the United States in 1994 and 1995 and detection of beta-lactamase–positive strains resistant to amoxicillin-clavulanate: results of a national multicenter surveillance study. Antimicrob Agents Chemother 41:292-297

18. Doern GV, Brueggemann AB, Pierce G, Hogan T, Holley HP Jr, Rauch A (1997) Prevalence of antimicrobial resistance among 723 outpatient clinical isolates of *Moraxella catarrhalis* in the United States in 1994 and 1995: Results of a 30-center national surveillance study. Antimicrob Agents Chemother 40:884-2886

19. Clavo-Sánchez AJ, Girón-González JA, López-Prieto D, et al. (1997) Multivariate analysis of risk factors for infection due to penicillin-resistant and multidrug-resistant *Streptococcus pneumoniae*: a multicenter study. Clin Infect Dis 24:1052-1059

20. Ewig S, Ruiz M, Torres A, Marco F, Martinez JA, Sanchez M, Mensa J (1999) Pneumonia acquired in the community through drug-resistant *Streptococcus pneumoniae*. Am J Respir Crit Care Med 159:1835-1842

21. Eller J, Ede A, Schaberg T, Niederman MS, Mauch H, Lode H (1998) Infective exacerbations of chronic bronchitis: Relation between bacteriologic etiology and lung function. Chest 113:1542-1548

22. Miravitlles M, Espinosa C, Fernandez-Laso E, Martos JA, Maldonado JA, Gallego M, et al. (1999) Relationship between bacterial flora in sputum and functional impairment in patients with acute exacerbations of COPD. Chest 116:40-46
23. Mandell LA (1994) Antibiotics for pneumonia therapy. Med Clin North Am 78:997-1014
24. Niederman MS (1997) The principles of antibiotic use and the selection of empiric therapy for pneumonia. In: Fishman A (ed) Pulmonary diseases and disorders, 3rd edn. McGraw-Hill, New York, pp 1939-1949
25. Niederman MS (1998) Treatment of respiratory infections with quinolones. In: Andriole V (ed) The quinolones, 2nd edn. Academic Press, San Diego, pp 229-250
26. Preston SL, Drusano GL, Berman AL, Fowler CL, Chow AT, Dornseif B, Reichl V, Natarajan J, Corrado M (1998) Pharmacodynamics of levofloxacin: a new paradigm for early clinical trials. JAMA 279:125-129
27. Anzueto A, Niederman MS, Tillotson GS, and the Bronchitis Study Group (1998) Etiology, susceptibility, and treatment of acute bacterial exacerbations of complicated chronic bronchitis in the primary care setting: Ciprofloxacin 750 mg BID vs clarithromycin 500 mg BID. Clin Ther 20(5):885-900
28. Chen DK, McGeer A, De Azavedo JC, Low DE, et al. (1999) Decreased susceptibility of *Streptococcus pneumoniae* to fluoroquinolones in Canada. N Engl J Med 341:233-239
29. Honeybourne D (1994) Antibiotic penetration into lung tissues. Thorax 49:104-106
30. Sonnesyn SW, Gerding DN (1994) Antimicrobials for the treatment of respiratory infection. In: Niederman MS, Sarosi GA, Glassroth J (eds) Respiratory infections: a scientific basis for management. WB Saunders, Philadelphia, pp 511-537
31. Gantz N (1990) Patient compliance in the management of adult respiratory infections. Intern Med Specialist 1990(10):1-3
32. Gallup Organization (1995) Consumer attitudes toward antibiotic use. American Lung Association, New York
33. Destache CJ, Dewan N, O'Donahue WJ, Campbell JC, Angelillo VA (1999) Clinical and economic considerations in the treatment of acute exacerbations of chronic bronchitis. J Antimicrob Chemother 43(Suppl A):107-113
34. Quenzer RW, Pettit KG, Arnold RJ, Kaniecki DJ (1997) Pharmacoeconomic analysis of selected antibiotics in lower respiratory tract infection. Am J Manag Care 3:1027-1036
35. Grossman R, Mukherjee M, Vaughan D, Eastwood C, Cook R, LaForge J, et al. (1998) A 1-year community-based health economic study of ciprofloxacin vs. usual antibiotic treatment in acute exacerbations of chronic bronchitis: The Canadian Ciprofloxacin Health Economic Study Group. Chest 113:131-141

Designing Future Clinical Trials
for Acute Exacerbations of Chronic Bronchitis

M. Miravitlles

Introduction

To some extent, chronic bronchitis can be considered an orphan disease. In fact, most (if not all) of the drugs used in the stable phase of the disease have been initially developed for treating asthma. Similarly, most trials aimed at demonstrating the efficacy of antibiotics in acute exacerbations (AECB) have been modelled on pneumonia studies. Research in both asthma and pneumonia has been the inspiration of subsequent studies in chronic bronchitis in many cases. Furthermore, a specific approach to the disease which takes into account its unique characteristics has seldom been used by researchers.

The definition of chronic bronchitis itself demonstrates the lack of interest in the disease over the last four decades. Unlike other chronic respiratory conditions such as bronchial asthma, of which the definition is periodically updated, the definition of chronic bronchitis does not include any reference to etiology, pathogenesis, pathology, signs, prognosis, etc. Its ambiguity hampers the design of clinical trials, since it permits the inclusion of a wide spectrum of patients with very different underlying pulmonary diseases and severities. Furthermore, there is no universally accepted definition of AECB, although the definition proposed by Anthonisen and coworkers [1], based on the number of symptoms present, is the most widely used. All these peculiarities imply that the interpretation of results of clinical trials on AECB is often confusing or inconclusive.

Characteristics of Existing Clinical Trials on Chronic Bronchitis

Antibiotics are significantly better than placebo for treating acute exacerbations of chronic obstructive pulmonary disease (COPD), i.e. in the treatment of

Servei de Pneumologia, Hospital General Vall d'Hebron, Barcelona, Spain patients with significant baseline airflow obstruction [1-3]. Antibiotics are particularly effective in patients presenting with more severe exacerbations in terms of number of symptoms at onset [1]. However, no study so far has demonstrated the superiority of antibiotics versus placebo in patients with "simple" chronic bronchitis, i.e. without airflow obstruction. Furthermore, some studies suggest that antibiotics add no benefit over a short course of oral corticosteroids in mild patients with exacerbated chronic bronchitis [4]. Consequently, there is a general agreement that antibiotics should be prescribed in exacerbations of chronic bronchitis in patients with chronic airflow limitation and especially if they present with two or more of the following symptoms: increasing dyspnea, increasing sputum production or increasing purulence of sputum (type 1 and 2 exacerbations). Conversely, antibiotics offer no benefit to patients without airflow obstruction, particularly if the exacerbation presents with only one of the previous symptoms (type 3). However, some confusion arises when the results of Anthonisen, et al. [1] and Allegra, et al. [2] are erroneously extrapolated to the complete spectrum of patients with chronic bronchitis. Therefore, antibiotics are recommended based exclusively on the number of symptoms at presentation, regardless of the severity of the underlying disease. It is necessary to keep in mind that patients in the Canadian study had moderate to severe COPD with a mean forced expiratory volume in 1 second (FEV_1) of 33% predicted, while the mean FEV_1 of patients in the Italian study was only 1.53 liters. Therefore, these results may not apply to patients with normal or near-normal pulmonary function, even if they present a type 1 or 2 exacerbation.

Considering the results of the last studies, together with the meta-analysis of Saint, et al. [3], it is difficult to undertake placebo-controlled trials in AECB based on ethical considerations. Most studies of antibiotics on AECB are randomized controlled trials of the newer antibiotics versus "standard agents", usually for registration purposes. These studies are designed to show equivalence in efficacy and safety with standard therapy. They include patients based on the only diagnostic criterion of "daily production of sputum on most days for at least 3 consecutive months for more than 2 consecutive years" [5-7] or with small modifications [8]. Not surprisingly, the mean age of patients in such studies is approximately 50-60 with a range from 18 to 90 years [5]. Some studies include as much as 24% of life-long non-smokers [6], and in one study which showed the range of pulmonary function impairment, the FEV_1 values were between 0.4 and 6.3 liters [8]. This again gives us an idea of the extremely imprecise definition of chronic bronchitis.

The majority of clinical trials exclude patients with significant comorbidity. This factor, together with the inclusion of young individuals with preserved ventilatory function, does not allow us to demonstrate the differences among cure rates of "traditional" antibiotics and newer antibiotics that are supposed to be more active. The reason is that milder patients without risk factors will recover spontaneously, regardless of the antibiotic prescribed [1, 4].

The outcome measures more widely used in existing clinical trials are the clinical and bacteriological responses obtained. Clinical results are evaluated as the remission of presenting symptoms, based on the personal subjective criterion of the investigator. Bacteriological results are based on the findings of sputum cultures. Usually, assessment of outcomes is performed at test-of-cure (5-10 days after starting therapy) and at follow-up (15-30 days after initiating the treatment). This design allows the demonstration of equivalence among different antibiotics, but is clearly insufficient to show differences in outcomes among different antimicrobial agents.

Designing New Trials for AECB

Developments in antimicrobial therapy have led to new generations of antibiotics with an extended spectrum of action. They are active against bacteria resistant to older traditional antibiotics and have improved pharmacokinetics and pharmacodynamics and powerful bactericidal actions. The introduction of these agents in the market should have an impact on the management of AECB; however, their superiority is still far from being proved in a clinical setting. Studies aimed at demonstrating such differences must be carefully designed considering the existing knowledge on pathophysiology of exacerbations.

Inclusion Criteria

Results of ambulatory treatment of AECB are far from optimal; observational studies have demonstrated a failure rate of 15%-25% [9-13]. Since the rate of failure in clinical trials oscillates between 8% and 12% [5-8], there must be some factors accounting for this difference. The most likely are the systematic exclusion of patients with either significant comorbidity or advanced age from clinical trials and the careful monitoring of compliance with medication. Ball, et al. [11] observed that major cardiopulmonary disease was a significant risk factor for returning to the general practitioner (GP) with a chest problem after being treated for AECB. Other identified risk factors for failure of ambulatory treatment of AECB were the number of previous AECB [7, 11, 14], the number of previous relapses [14], a history of prolonged chronic bronchitis [7], and a reduced FEV_1 [14] or FEV_1/FVC ratio [8]. All these variables are related to either the past history of the disease or the patient's baseline characteristics. Surprisingly, the severity of the presenting exacerbation, classified by the number of symptoms, does not seem to influence outcome in most studies [7, 11, 14]. A list of possible severity markers for chronic bronchitis is displayed in Table 1 [7, 8, 14-20].

The mentioned studies provide valuable information about which patients are more likely to relapse. Therefore, better designed antibiotics, if properly assessed, should offer improved results in this selected, more severely affected population. Table 2 summarizes the desirable inclusion criteria for studies

Table 1. Severity markers for chronic bronchitis

At baseline
  Low FEV_1 and/or low FEV_1/FVC ratio
  Impaired score on dyspnea scales
  Low pO_2
  Impaired score in HRQL questionnaires
  Low body mass index (BMI)
  Impaired 6-minute walking test

Historic
  More than 3 previous medical visits for chest problems in the past year
  More than 3 acute exacerbations in the previous year
  Coexisting chronic conditions (especially cardiopulmonary)
  Chronic mucus hypersecretion

FEV_1, mean forced expiratory volume in 1 second; *FVC*, forced vital capacity, *HRQL*, health-related quality of life

Table 2. Criteria for new clinical trials in exacerbations of chronic bronchitis

Exclusion criteria
  "Only" chronic bronchitis
  Low score of symptoms at baseline
  History of type 3 exacerbations
  Life-long non-smokers

Inclusion criteria
  $FEV_1 < 50\%$ predicted
  High score of symptoms at baseline
  Type 1 or 2 exacerbations
  History of bacterial AECB (sputum culture positive)

FEV1, mean forced expiratory volume in 1 second; *AECB*, acute exacerbations of chronic bronchitis

aimed to demonstrate superiority between different antibiotics. Life-long non-smokers should not be included because their respiratory symptoms must be related to other underlying respiratory diseases such as bronchiectasis, and often need more extensive diagnostic investigation and a different therapeutic approach. An FEV_1 below 50% predicted has been chosen because, in addition to their worse prognosis, a recent study demonstrated that exacerbations in these patients are more frequently associated with significant bacterial growth in sputum [21].

Outcome Measures

Studies based exclusively on the clinical outcome "cure" or "improvement" are no longer acceptable. These variables are subject to the interpretation of the investigator. Thus, multicenter studies with many different investigators from different countries may interpret clinical results in a different sense. It is generally agreed that clinical assessment is necesary; however, it should be standardized and quantified. Allegra, et al. [2] proposed a score of symptoms and signs which included 6 different and readily-obtainable variables; by adding the subtotals of all 6 items, a final score ranging from 0 to 18 is obtained, with a difference of more than 3 points being considered clinically significant. This could be a starting point for the development of a quantified, standardized questionnaire similar to the health-related quality of life questionnaires already developed for clinical practice. The introduction of such questionnaires should minimize subjective interpretation of symptoms and allow comparisons of effects using the magnitude of the difference between pre- and post-antibiotic treatment with different agents. Nevertheless, clinical response should not be the only "clinical" outcome. Unlike pneumonia, AECB always occurs in a host with an underlying disease. Furthermore, as has already been mentioned, characteristics of the underlying disease are the main predictors of the outcome; therefore, determination of baseline characteristics of the patients should be paramount. In this sense, studies on AECB should be modelled after asthma, which is also a chronic respiratory disease with periods of increased symptoms. To obtain reliable data of the baseline conditions, patients should be enrolled while in stable phase and be followed, ideally for not less than one year, to obtain other outcome measures related to time to baseline or relapse.

The inclusion of time as an outcome variable has a solid scientific background. Although symptoms of exacerbation develop over a short period of time, some evidence suggests that the course of the exacerbation is subacute and the inflammatory processes that acompany the clinical manifestations may start weeks before symptoms appear. Murata, et al. [22] observed that some patients suffered a decrease in peak flow during the weeks preceeding the clinical manifestations of AECB. This observation is in agreement with the hypothesis that a certain bacterial load in the lower airways is needed for symptoms to develop. Monsó and coworkers [23] observed that a significant number of stable COPD patients had bacteria in their lower airways without clinical symptoms of exacerbation. However, the number of patients carrying bacteria increased significantly during exacerbations. Furthermore, exacerbated patients had higher bacterial counts than stable patients, thus supporting the theory of the bacterial load. Also, a recent study demonstrated that bronchial colonization with potentially pathogenic microorganisms in COPD may represent an independent stimulus for additional airway inflammation [24]. Similarly, after the clinical resolution of symptoms, inflammation in the airways may still persist, as shown in an elegant study by Agustí, et al. [25]. They demonstrated that the elevated exhaled nitric oxide levels in patients with exacerbation did not return to normal until several months later. A very recent study has described the time course of various inflammatory markers, both in plasma and sputum, during an exacerbation of COPD [26]. It demonstrated that C-reactive protein (CRP) is a good marker in blood [26, 27], and that myeloperoxidase (MPO), interleukin-8 (IL-8) and leukotriene B4 (LTB4) are useful markers of the course of exacerbation in sputum [26]. The levels of these proteins are elevated during exacerbations and decrease rapidly with 14 days of antibiotic treatment. The possibility of differences in magnitude, or speed of recovery, of all these parameters with the use of different antibiotics should be further explored.

The next clinical parameter to be used as an outcome is pulmonary function. A transient impairment in pulmonary function during exacerbations has been observed in most studies [1, 2, 6]. In one study, the speed of recovery of peak expiratory flow (PEF) was significantly faster in patients treated with antibiotics compared to placebo [1], whereas in another study FEV_1 values returned to baseline after antibiotic treatment but not after placebo [2]. It is possible that in severely affected patients, speed or intensity of recovery of PEF or FEV_1, or both, may show significant differences between treatments with different antimicrobials.

The development of standardized and validated health-related quality of life (HRQL) questionnaires has permitted the quantification of the impact of disease on patients' general well-being. Some disease-specific questionnaires have been demonstrated to be useful in identifying patients more at risk of relapse of exacerbation in a cohort of severely affected COPD patients [15]. Such questionnaires are being extensively used in clinical trials with drugs such as bronchodilators or inhaled corticosteroids used for long-term treatment in COPD; in addition, they have also provided useful information in placebo-controlled studies of oral corticosteroids in acute exacerbations of COPD [28]. This latter study showed that St. George's Respiratory Questionnaire (SGRQ) scores were, in most cases, still abnormal six weeks after the exacerbation. Therefore, time to baseline scores in HRQL questionnaires is another outcome that can be used to show differences among different treatments. These questionnaires have been seldom used in trials with antibiotics; however, Grossman, et al. [7] observed that results in terms of HRQL were different in comparing different antibiotic regimens for exacerbations of COPD. The differences were more evident in patients with more risk factors for poor evolution of the exacerbation.

Repeated exacerbations have been shown to significantly impair HRQL of COPD patients [29]. If an antibiotic is able to prolong the symptom-free interval, it will be expected to preserve the HRQL of patients. Thus, HRQL scores may be used in long-term follow-up of patients to illustrate the impact of recurrent exacerbations and the possible beneficial effects of new antibiotics.

The possible deleterious effect of recurrent or persistent bronchial infection on lung parenchyma or bronchi is under debate. At present, there is not enough evidence of accelerated loss of lung function due to recurrent infection or colonization of the lower airways, especially because studies aimed to demonstrate such effect are hampered by the slow progession of impairment and the great interindividual variability of rate of decline. Nevertheless, there is increasing evidence that colonization of the lower airways is associated with increased inflammatory responses and is inversely correlated with FEV_1 [24, 30]. When bacterial load increases, recruitment of secondary host defenses will result in an increase in airway inflammation and neutrophil influx. As a result of activated metabolism of neutrophils, there is an increase in free neutrophil elastase and oxidants which have the potential to cause harmful effects on lung parenchyma and airways [31]. This has been clearly demonstrated in the form of early-onset emphysema [26] or bronchiectasis [32] in patients with alpha-1 proteinase inhibitor deficiency. However, this effect may be occurring to a lesser extent in patients with normal concentrations of the inhibitor. Since pulmonary function tests are insensitive in detecting these changes in small populations over a short period of time, new techniques must be developed to quantify the possible deleterious effects of recurrent lung infection. A recent study suggested that quantitation of emphysema by computed tomography (CT) is more than twice as sensitive for detecting the progression of lung parenchymal lesions than pulmonary function tests [33]. The use of this technique in the long-term follow-up of patients with recurrent AECB may be of value in detecting the pernicious effects of infection on the lungs. Also, due to its high sensitivity it may be useful in illustrating differences between antibiotic options in the future.

Another important aspect of antibiotic treatment of AECB is the pharmacoeconomic analysis [34]. Antibiotics account for only 15%-20% of the total direct costs of AECB [9]; consequently, a new, more expensive antibiotic can be cost-effective by showing a small reduction in treatment failures. By using a pharmacoeconomic approach, a recent study showed that a more expensive antibiotic was cost-effective in the treatment of AECB in high risk patients [7].

Finally, bacteriological assessment is required in such clinical trials. Ideally, uncontaminated samples from the lower respiratory tract are desireable. This approach has been successfully used in severe exacerbated COPD patients admitted to intensive care units [35]. However, the practice of invasive microbiological diagnostic techniques in a large scale study in an ambulatory setting is unrealistic. The study of sputum samples with its intrinsic limitations would be the technique of choice, and the assessment of bacterial eradication, persistence or relapse would be the main outcomes. Bacterial and clinical results usually correlate; however, clinical success despite bacterial persistence has been well documented [6]. There are many possible reasons for this discrepancy, one being the presence of different strains of the same microorganism with different antimicrobial susceptibilities [36]. It can therefore be hypothesized that a given antibiotic would kill those susceptible bacteria, decreasing the bacterial load enough to decrease inflammation and relieve symptoms, but resistant bacteria would survive. While the differences in eradication rates of two antibiotics have not been demonstrated to influence the rate of relapse, time to relapse, loss of HRQL, increased lung damage or any other clinical parameter, and while bacterial persistence in the airways has not been undoubtedly demonstrated to damage the lung, both antibiotics must be regarded as equally effective, since what really matters is the clinical outcome of the patient, not the bacteria.

Comparators and Concomitant Medication

Antibiotics used as comparators in clinical trials with new antimicrobials must fulfil some characteristics: (a) they must be indicated for treatment of AECB; (b) they must have the same route of administration, usually oral; and (c) they must be widely used in the community. The important aspect of such new trials would be the demonstration of superiority of new antibiotics over the traditional, so-called first-line agents. We must keep in mind that there is a huge number of different antibiotics used in the community [12] and some of the so-called first-line agents (amoxicillin, doxycycline or trimethoprim-sulfamethoxazole) are almost not being used in some countries at present [37]. It would not make any sense to demonstrate the superiority against antibiotics that are not used for this indication anymore. Comparison should be made among the most prescribed antimicrobials: amoxicillin-clavulanate, clarithromycin, azythromycin, cefuroxime axetil and the new fluoroquinolones.

A short course of oral corticosteroids has been shown to be superior to placebo for the clinical resolution of symptoms of AECB [28, 38, 39]. Therefore, the use of oral corticosteroids must be controlled in such trials. Based on the existing evidence, it is difficult to justify not prescribing corticosteroids in AECB, thus all groups of patients should receive them. However, it would be relevant to compare corticosteroids alone and corticosteroids with antibiotics in a double-blind trial. The possible trial could be: *group a,* corticosteroid plus placebo; *group b,* corticosteroids plus antibiotic I; and *group c,* corticosteroids plus antibiotic II.

The Ideal Clinical Trial

The need for new clinical trials to demonstrate differences among antibiotics in the treatment of AECB has been largely recognized [40]; however, no standard clinical trial has been designed yet. A possible starting point is presented in Table 3. Of course, the complexity and duration of the trial must be in accordance with the possible resources. Also, other parameters may be added following new technical developments or relevant scientific findings. The proposal is only intended to be a possible basis for future research and development.

With the use of strict inclusion criteria and different clinical, microbiological, biochemical and imaging outcomes, it should be possible to demonstrate relevant differences among antibiotics for the treatment of AECB if they really exist.

Table 3. Project for a clinical trial to demonstrate significant differences in outcomes of AECB among tested antibiotics

Screen patients in stable phase following inclusion and exclusion criteria (Table 2)
Determine baseline characteristics:
  Clinical
    Symptoms score
    Pulmonary function tests
    HRQL
    Six-minute walking test

  Biochemical
    NO in exhaled air
    CRP in plasma
    IL-8, LTB-4, MPO, elastase in sputum

  Imaging
    Lung density by CT

At exacerbation:
  Repeat full assessment, except CT
  Microbiological analysis of sputum

Control visits at days 1, 3, 5, 7, 14, 28 after exacerbation
  At all visits
    Symptoms score
    Pulmonary function tests
    Biochemical markers
    Microbiological analysis of sputum

  At visits 7, 14, 28
    HRQL

Follow-up visits every month for at least one year. Perform all tests until return to baseline:
  Symptoms score
  Pulmonary function tests
  Biochemical markers
  Microbiological analysis of sputum
  HRQL
If new exacerbation occurs, record time free of symptoms.

Last visit at least 12 months after exacerbation
  Symptoms score
  Pulmonary function tests
  HRQL
  Lung density by CT
  Pharmacoeconomic analysis

HRQL, health-related quality of life; *NO,* nitric oxide; *CRP,* C-reactive protein; *IL-8,* interleukin-8; *LTB4,* leukotriene B4; *MPO,* myeloperoxidase; *CT,* computed tomography

References

1. Anthonisen NR, Manfreda J, Warren CPW, Hershfield ES, Harding GKM, Nelson NA (1987) Antibiotic therapy in exacerbations of chronic obstructive pulmonary disease. Ann Intern Med 106:196-204
2. Allegra L, Grassi C, Grossi E, Pozzi E, Blasi F, Frigerio D, et al. (1991) Ruolo degli antibiotici nel trattamento delle riacutizzazioni della bronchite cronica: risultati di uno studio italiano multicentrico. Ital J Chest Dis 45:138-148
3. Saint S, Bent S, Vittinghoff E, Grady D (1995) Antibiotics in chronic obstructive pulmonary disease exacerbations: a meta-analysis. JAMA 273:957-960
4. Sachs APE, Köter GH, Groenier KH, van der Waaij D, Schiphuis J, Meyboom-de Jong B (1995) Changes in symptoms, peak expiratory flow, and sputum flora during treatment with antibiotics of exacerbations in patients with chronic obstructive pulmonary disease in general practice. Thorax 50:758-763
5. Chodosh S, DeAbate CA, Haverstock D, Aneiro L, Church D and the Bronchitis Study Group (2000) Short-course moxifloxacin therapy for treatment of acute bacterial exacerbations of chronic bronchitis. Respir Med 94:18-27
6. Wilson R, Kubin R, Ballin I, Deppermann KM, Bassaris HP, Leophonte P, et al. (1999) Five day moxifloxacin therapy compared with 7 day clarithromycin therapy for the treatment of acute exacerbations of chronic bronchitis. J Antimicrob Chemother 44:501-513
7. Grossman R, Mukherjee J, Vaughan D, Eastwood C, Cook R, LaForge J, et al. (1998) A 1-year community-based health economic study of ciprofloxacin vs usual antibiotic treatment in acute exacerbations of chronic bronchitis. Chest 113:131-141
8. DeAbate CA, Henry D, Bensch G, Jubran A, Chodosh S, Harper L, et al. (1998) Sparfloxacin vs ofloxacin in the treatment of acute bacterial exacerbations of chronic bronchitis. A multicenter, double-blind, randomized, comparative study Chest 114:120-130
9. Miravitlles M, Murio C, Guerrero T, Segú JL (1999) Costs derived from management of acute exacerbations of chronic bronchitis and COPD. Eur Respir J 14 (Suppl 30):115s
10. MacFarlane JT, Colville A, Guion A, MacFarlane RM, Rose DH (1993) Prospective study of aetiology and outcome of adult lower respiratory tract infections in the community. Lancet 341:511-514
11. Ball P, Harris JM, Lowson D, Tillotson G, Wilson R (1995) Acute infective exacerbations of chronic bronchitis. Q J Med 88:61-68
12. Huchon GJ, Gialdroni-Grassi G, Léophonte P, Manresa F, Schaberg T, Woodhead M (1996) Initial antibiotic therapy for lower respiratory tract infection in the community: a European survey. Eur Respir J 9:1590-1595
13. Davey P, Rutherford D, Graham B, Lynch B, Malek M (1994) Repeat consultations after antibiotic prescribing for respiratory infection: a study in one general practice. Br J Gen Pract 44:509-513
14. Murata GH, Gorby MS, Kapsner CO, Chick TW, Halperin AK (1992) A multivariate model for predicting hospital admissions for patients with decompensated chronic obstructive pulmonary disease. Arch Intern Med 152:82-86
15. Osman LM, Godden DJ, Friend JAR, Legge JS, Douglas JG (1997) Quality of life and hospital re-admission in patients with chronic obstructive pulmonary disease. Thorax 52:67-71
16. Antonelli Incalzi R, Fuso L, De Rosa M, Forastiere F, Rapiti E, Nardecchia B, et al. (1997) Co-morbidity contributes to predict mortality of patients with chronic obstructive pulmonary disease. Eur Respir J 10:2794-2800

17. Prescott E, Lange P, Vestbo J (1995) Chronic mucus hypersecretion in COPD and death from pulmonary infection. Eur Respir J 8:1333-1338
18. Landbo C, Prescott E, Lange P, Vestbo J, Almidal TP (1999) Prognostic value of nutritional status in chronic obstructive pulmonary disease. Am J Respir Crit Care Med 160:1856-1861
19. Kessler R, Faller M, Fourgaut G, Mennecier B, Weitzenblum E (1999) Predictive factors of hospitalization for acute exacerbation in a series of 64 patients with chronic obstructive pulmonary disease. Am J Respir Crit Care Med 159:158-164
20. Connors AF Jr, Dawson NV, Thomas C, Harrel FE Jr, Desbiens N, Fulkerson WJ, et al. (1996) Outcomes following acute exacerbation of severe chronic obstructive pulmonary disease. Am J Respir Crit Care Med 154:959-967
21. Miravitlles M, Espinosa C, Fernández-Laso E, Martos JA, Maldonado JA, Gallego M and Study Group of Bacterial Infection in COPD (1999) Relationship between bacterial flora in sputum and functional impairment in patients with acute exacerbations of COPD. Chest 116: 40-46.
22. Murata GH, Kapsner CO, Lium DJ, Busby HK (1998) Time course of respiratory decompensation in chronic obstructive pulmonary disease: a prospective, double-blind study of peak flow changes prior to emergency department visit. Respir Med 92:936-941
23. Monsó E, Ruiz J, Rosell A, Monterola J, Fiz J, Morera J, Ausina V (1995) Bacterial infection in chronic obstructive pulmonary disease. A study of stable and exacerbated outpatients using the protected specimen brush. Am J Respir Crit Care Med 152:1316-1320
24. Soler N, Ewig S, Torres A, Filella X, Gonzalez J, Xaubet A (1999) Airway inflammation and bronchial microbial patterns in patients with stable chronic obstructive pulmonary disease. Eur Respir J 14:1015-1022
25. Agustí AGN, Villaverde JM, Togores B, Bosch M (1999) Serial measurements of exhaled nitric oxide during exacerbations of chronic obstructive pulmonary disease. Eur Respir J 14:523-528
26. Hill AT, Campbell EJ, Bayley DL, Hill SL, Stockley RA (1999) Evidence for excessive bronchial inflammation during an acute exacerbation of chronic obstructive pulmonary disease in patients with alpha-1-antitrypsin deficiency (PiZ). Am J Respir Crit Care Med 160:1968-1975
27. Dev D, Wallace E, Sankaran R, Cunnife J, Govan JRW, Wathen CG, et al. (1998) Value of C-reactive protein measurements in exacerbations of chronic obstructive pulmonary disease. Respir Med 92:664-667
28. Davies L, Angus RM, Calverley PMA (1999) Oral corticosteroids in patients admitted to hospital with exacerbations of chronic obstructive pulmonary disease: a prospective randomised controlled trial. Lancet 354:456-460
29. Seemungal TAR, Donaldson GC, Paul EA, Bestall JC, Jeffries DJ, Wedzicha JA (1998) Effect of exacerbation on quality of life in patients with chronic obstructive pulmonary disease. Am J Respir Crit Care Med 157:1418-1422
30. Di Stefano A, Capelli A, Lusuardi M, Balbo P, Vecchio C, Maestrelli P, et al. (1998) Severity of airflow limitation is associated with severity of airway inflammation in smokers. Am J Respir Crit Care Med 158:1277-1285
31. Stockley RA (1998) Role of bacteria in the pathogenesis and progression of acute and chronic lung infection. Thorax 53:58-62
32. Miravitlles M, de Gracia J, Rodrigo MJ, Cruz MJ, Vendrell M, Vidal R, et al. (1999) Specific antibody response against the 23-valent pneumococcal vaccine in patients with alpha-1-antitrypsin deficiency with and without bronchiectasis. Chest 116:946-952

33. Dirksen A, Dijkman JH, Madsen F, Stoel B, Hutchinson DCS, Ulrik CS, et al. (1999) A randomized clinical trial of alpha-1-antitrypsin augmentation therapy. Am J Respir Crit Care Med 160:1468-1472

34. Davey PG, Malek MM, Parker SE (1992) Pharmacoeconomics of antibacterial treatment. Pharmacoeconomics 1:409-437

35. Soler N, Torres A, Ewig S, Gonzalez J, Celis R, El-Ebiary M, et al. (1998) Bronchial microbial patterns in severe exacerbations of chronic obstructive pulmonary disease (COPD) requiring mechanical ventilation. Am J Respir Crit Care Med 157:1498-1505

36. Murphy TF, Sethi S, Klingman KL, Brueggemann AB, Doern GV (1999) Simultaneous respiratory tract colonization by multiple strains of nontypeable haemophilus influenzae in chronic obstructive pulmonary disease: implications from antibiotic therapy. J Infect Dis 180:404-409

37. Miravitlles M, Mayordomo C, Artés M, Sánchez-Agudo L, Nicolau F, Segú JL on behalf of the EOLO Group (1999) Treatment of chronic obstructive pulmonary disease and its exacerbations in general practice. Respir Med 93:173-179

38. Thompson WH, Nielson CP, Carvalho P, Charan N, Crowley J (1996) Controlled trial of oral prednisone in outpatients with acute COPD exacerbations. Am J Respir Crit Care Med 154:407-412.

39. Niewoehner DE, Erbland ML, Deupree RH, Collins D, Gross NJ, Light RW, et al. (1999) Effect of systemic glucocorticoids on exacerbations of chronic obstructive pulmonary disease. N Engl J Med 340:1941-1947

40. Wilson R, Tillotson G, Ball P (1996) Clinical studies in chronic bronchitis: a need for a better definition and classification of severity. J Antimicrob Chemother 37:205-207

Perspectives and Perceptions
on the Management of Acute Exacerbations of COPD

L. ALLEGRA, F. BLASI

Chronic obstructive pulmonary disease (COPD) is present in 20% of the population in the United States [1]. The development of the disease involves multiple risk factors including genetic predisposition, maternal smoking, nutrition, allergens, active and passive smoking, infection, air pollution, etc. In the past decades two major theories have been put forward to explain the pathogenesis of chronic bronchitis. The Dutch and the British hypotheses have generally been considered competing theories, the first underscoring the importance of hyperreactivity, the latter the role of infection [2, 3]. However, as suggested by Rennard, the underlying process is an upsetting of the tissue damage/tissue repair balance that initiates inflammatory derangement directly leading to airway remodelling and airflow obstruction [4].

In this context, exacerbations of chronic bronchitis are a common occurrence in clinical practice, and are a leading cause of antibiotic prescription among respiratory infections. It is still uncertain whether each new exacerbation may deteriorate the natural history of chronic bronchitis. Undoubtedly, every episode induces a temporary worsening in lung function and may therefore pose a threat of respiratory failure or death in more severely obstructed patients.

Exacerbations are traditionally defined as an increase in cough, a change in the color or quantity of sputum, or worsening dyspnea [5]. Although clinically descriptive, the above definition is of little practical use in identifying prognostic and treatment factors in individual patients. In his chapter in the present book, Peter Ball indicates the possible application of a new, simple classification to identify patients in whom antibiotic treatment is indicated. Recognizing specific risk factors predictive of poor response to treatment may prove a further valuable aid in deciding appropriate treatment of exacerbations.

Underlying disease severity preceding exacerbations has been recognized as an important factor, since bacterial etiology of exacerbations is predictable on the basis of the degree of functional derangement. Correct etiological identification

Institute of Respiratory Diseases, University of Milan, IRCCS Ospedale Maggiore, Milan, Italy of single exacerbations is therefore important in defining patient natural history. As underlined in the chapter by Chodosh, microbiological sputum analysis is therefore still a fundamental diagnostic tool, providing fulfilment of stringent collection and microscopic evaluation criteria. It has been shown that the results of diagnostic evaluation caused a change in antimicrobial treatment in over one-third of patients with severe COPD exacerbations [6]. In addition to the more complex microbiological pattern of severe COPD exacerbations, problems are now encountered in the treatment of exacerbations of patients with mild COPD due to increasing resistance patterns among typical pathogens such as *Streptococcus pneumoniae.*

Correct antibiotic treatment plays a central role in conditioning the outcome of exacerbations and may influence the natural history of the disease. The utility of antibiotic therapy has now fairly definitively been demonstrated [7] and the characteristics of the ideal antimicrobial have been neatly summed up by Niederman: efficacy towards most common and likely pathogens; resistance to destruction by beta-lactamases; good pharmacodynamic properties; and cost effectiveness.

Considering that comparisons between new antimicrobial agents and placebo are no longer ethically acceptable, future clinical pharmacology trials must demonstrate superiority towards existing agents. As indicated in the chapter by Miravitlles, future studies will have to include a complete clinical and functional assessment of patients in steady state, re-evaluation during exacerbation, and follow-up at at least one year. Quality of life and pharmaco-economic parameters are also mandatory for the complete evaluation of an antibiotic treatment.

References

1. American Thoracic Society (1995) Standards for the diagnosis and care of patients with chronic obstructive pulmonary disease. Am J Respir Crit Care Med 152:S77-S120
2. Weiss ST, Speizer FE (1984) Increased level of airways responsiveness as a risk factor for development of chronic obstructive lung disease: what are the issues? Chest 86:3
3. Fletcher C, Peto R, Tinker C, Speizer FE (1976) The natural history of chronic bronchitis and emphysema. Oxford University, Oxford
4. Rennard SI (1998) COPD: overview of definitions, epidemiology, and factors influencing its development. Chest 113:235S-241S
5. Anthonisen NR, Manfreda J, Warren CPW, Hershfield ES, Harding GKM, Nelson NA (1987) Antibiotic therapy in exacerbations of chronic obstructive pulmonary disease. Ann Intern Med 106:196-204
6. Ewig S, Soler N, Gonzalez J, El-Ebiary M, Celis R, Torres A (2000) Evaluation of antimicrobial treatment in mechanically ventilated patients with severe COPD exacerbations. Crit Care Med (*in press*)
7. Saint S, Bent S, Vittinghoff E, Grady D (1995) Antibiotics in chronic obstructive pulmonary disease exacerbations. A meta-analysis. JAMA 273:957-960